Essential Orthodontics

Essential Orthodontics

Birgit Thilander
Former Professor Emerita, Odont Dr (PhD), DDS
Institute of Odontology
Sahlgrenska Academy
University of Gothenburg
Gothenburg
Sweden

Krister Bjerklin
Associate Professor, Odont Dr (PhD), DDS
Department of Orthodontics
The Institute for Postgraduate Dental Education in Jönköping
Jönköping
Sweden

Lars Bondemark
Professor, Odont Dr (PhD), DDS
Department of Orthodontics
Faculty of Odontology
Malmö University
Malmö
Sweden

WILEY Blackwell

Registered Offices: John Wiley & Sons, Inc., 111 River Street, Hoboken, NJ 07030, USA
John Wiley & Sons Ltd, The Atrium, Southern Gate, Chichester, West Sussex, PO19 8SQ, UK

Editorial Office: 9600 Garsington Road, Oxford, OX4 2DQ, UK

For details of our global editorial offices, customer services, and more information about Wiley products visit us at www.wiley.com.

Wiley also publishes its books in a variety of electronic formats and by print-on-demand. Some content that appears in standard print versions of this book may not be available in other formats.

Library of Congress Cataloging-in-Publication Data

Names: Thilander, Birgit, 1924–2016, author. | Bjerklin, Erik, 1946– author.
  | Bondemark, Lars, 1955– author.
Title: Essential orthodontics / Birgit Thilander, Erik Bjerklin, Lars
  Bondemark.
Description: First edition. | Hoboken, NJ : John Wiley & Sons, Inc., 2018. |
  Includes bibliographical references and index.
Identifiers: LCCN 2017009365 (print) | LCCN 2017010816 (ebook) | ISBN
  9781119165675 (pbk.) | ISBN 9781119165682 (pdf) | ISBN 9781119165699 (epub)
Subjects: | MESH: Orthodontics | Malocclusion | Biomechanical Phenomena
Classification: LCC RK521 (ebook) | LCC RK521 (print) | NLM WU 400 | DDC
  617.6/43–dc23
LC record available at https://lccn.loc.gov/2017010816

Cover Design: Wiley
Cover Image: Courtesy of Lars Bondemark

Set in 10/12pt, AGaramondPro-Regular by SPi Global, Chennai, India.
Printed and bound in Singapore by Markono Print Media Pte Ltd

10 9 8 7 6 5 4 3 2

Contents

List of Abbreviations

Acronym	Definition
ACF	alveolar-crest fibres
AF	apical fibres
ANB angle	sagittal skeletal inter jaw relation
BMP	bone morphogenetic protein
CBCT	Cone Beam Computered Tomography
CEJ	cement-enamel junction
CLP	cleft lip and palate
CT	computer tomography
Cx	transmembrane connexion
3D	Three-dimensional
DAI	Dental Aesthetic Index
DC/TMD	Diagnostic Criteria for Temporomandibular Disorders
DS	dental stages
DS 01	primary dentition erupting
DS 02	primary dentition complete
DS 1	early mixed dentition with incisors erupting
DS 2	mixed dentition with incisors fully erupted
DS 3	late mixed dentition with canines and premolars erupting
DS 4	permanent dentition with canines and premolars fully erupted
DS M0	first molars erupting
DS M1	first molars fully erupted
DS M2	second molars fully erupted
DS M3	third molars fully erupted
FGF	fibroblast growth factor
GF	gingival fibres
HF	horizontal fibres
ICON	Index of Complexity, Outcome and Need
ICP	intercuspal relationship/centric relationship
IL	interleukin
ILi/ML	mandibular incisor inclination
ILs/NL	maxillary incisor inclination
IOTN-AC	Index of Orthodontic Treatment Need Aesthetic Component

Acronym	Definition
IOTN-DHC	Index of Orthodontic Treatment Need Dental Health Component
ICP	intercuspal position
M-CSF	macrophage colony-stimulating factor
MIH	molar incisor hypomineralization
ML	mandibular line
NL	nasal line
NL/ML	skeletal vertical inter jaw relation
Nor HS	Index of Norwegian Health Service
NSL	nasion sella line/cranial base line
NSL/ML	vertical inclination of the mandible
OF	oblique fibres
OPG	osteoprotegerin
PAR	Peer Assessment Rating
PDL	periodontal ligament
PG	prostaglandin
PHV	peak height velocity
PZ	proliferating zone
RANKL	receptor activator of nuclear factor kappa-B ligand
RCT	randomised controlled trial
RF	interradicular fibres
RL	ramus line
RME	rapid maxillary expansion
RP	mandibular retroposition
SARME	surgically assisted rapid maxillary expansion
SBU	Swedish Agency for Health Technology Assessment and Assessment of Social Services
SD	standard deviation
SNA angle	sagittal skeletal relation of the maxilla
SNB angle	sagittal skeletal relation of the mandible
Swe NBH	Index of Swedish National Board of Health
TAD	temporary anchorage device
TGF-ß	transforming growth factor-ß
TMD	temporomandibular disorder
TMJ	temporomandibular joint
TNF-α	tumour necrosis factor alpha
TRAP	tartrate-resistant acid and phosphatase
WSL	white spot lesion

Preface

In a limited sense, orthodontics is the art and science of aligning malpositioned teeth but it also includes a subdiscipline, known as dentofacial orthopaedics. While orthodontics ordinarily involves the movement of teeth in relation to the supporting structures, dentofacial orthopaedics aims at changing the interrelationship between the jaws. The borderline between these types has become somewhat diffuse, as morphological changes and tissue reactions associated with them show a great deal of overlap. The aim of this book is to discuss the principles of treatment planning, based on differential diagnosis as well as the biological stage of the individual (children in mixed/permanent dentition, adolescents, adults) to give a modern concept of orthodontics. Today, a wide variety of therapeutic techniques is available with special preferences in the different technique programmes, but they will not be described in detail in this book.

Orthodontics has changed its character during the last decades due to intense basic research on craniofacial growth and tissue response to orthodontic/orthopaedic forces, an explosive rate of development within the field of dental materials, a considerable improvement of dental health in many countries and increased social esteem afforded to orthodontic care. The treatment indication area has also widened, in that children as well as adults are increasingly subjected to orthodontic treatment. For the patient, an improvement of facial aesthetics of dentofacial anomalies is the reason for orthodontic therapy. Furthermore, orthodontics is increasingly regarded as an obvious component in the total dental plan, which has resulted in intensified collaboration and team-work between orthodontists and representatives of other disciplines. Thus, orthodontics today is a genuine art of the common health care.

It is the hope of the authors that, in addition to making the dental student familiar with the essentials of orthodontics, this book also may serve as a stimulus for further studies to those students who find orthodontics a discipline of special interest.

Birgit Thilander
Krister Bjerklin
Lars Bondemark

Acknowledgement

Professor Emerita Birgit Thilander, who passed away in the absolute final stage of completing the *Essential Orthodontics*, was the one who initiated this project. Her ultimate wish was that this book should be published.

It was a privilege to have had the opportunity to write the *Essential Orthodontics* together with Professor Thilander, who must be counted as one of the world's most famous researchers and teachers in orthodontics.

We remember with warmth a highly respected colleague and friend.

We are very grateful to Professor Maria Ransjö, who critically examined and brought fruitful comments and corrections to the text of Chapters 3 and 9, as well as parts of Chapter 11. We highly benefited from her expertise and efforts to help us present facts as correctly as possible.

Lars Bondemark and Krister Bjerklin

PART 1

Pretreatment Considerations

An adequate orthodontic diagnosis of our prospective patients, of all ages with different ethnic origins, is based on a systematic clinical examination, sound knowledge of classification of malocclusions and craniofacial growth and development.

Essential Orthodontics, First Edition. Birgit Thilander, Krister Bjerklin and Lars Bondemark.
© 2018 John Wiley & Sons Ltd. Published 2018 by John Wiley & Sons Ltd.

PART 1

Pretreatment
Considerations

CHAPTER 1
Orthodontic panorama

Birgit Thilander, Krister Bjerklin and Lars Bondemark

Key topics

- The orthodontic patient
- Individuals with different demands for orthodontic treatment
- Orthodontic care systems

Learning objectives

- To be able to handle individuals with orthodontic problems
- To understand what essential orthodontics implies

Essential Orthodontics, First Edition. Birgit Thilander, Krister Bjerklin and Lars Bondemark.
© 2018 John Wiley & Sons Ltd. Published 2018 by John Wiley & Sons Ltd.

Orthodontic panorama

Orthodontics is an old speciality that has undergone dramatic changes during the last 50 years, from being a discipline aimed at treating malocclusions in children to being a discipline aimed at treating patients irrespective of age. Who are then the prospective orthodontic patients? Where do they come from? Why do they come for treatment? Indeed, they make up a miscellaneous collection of individuals of varying ages, with different types of malocclusions, with different family histories, and with different social and cultural backgrounds, factors that naturally will influence the individual's response to orthodontic treatment strategies. Broadly speaking, they can be divided into the following categories that correspond with their special problems: children and teenagers, adults, children with cleft-lip-palate defects and children with disabilities.

The largest group consists of children and teenagers, about 70% of whom are estimated to have some type of malocclusion or tooth anomaly; however, this does not necessarily imply that all those individuals need orthodontic treatment. Treatment depends upon the anomaly, and some diagnosed at an early age have anomalies that may self-correct, while others can get worse. Therefore, it is important for regular examinations and check-ups during the dentofacial growth period, preferably starting at the early ages.

The development of dentition in the growing face is a complex process, as consequently there are many aspects of this process that can go wrong. It is thus of utmost importance that the general dentist is well up-to-date with a high level of knowledge of the classification of malocclusions and craniofacial growth and development. Nevertheless, it must be stressed that there are highly individual variations in dental and physical development, as well as in psychological maturity in children that deserve attention when performing an orthodontic procedure. For example, a treatment performed most effectively at an early age may involve another type of orthodontic procedure if postponed.

In most countries, the general dentist has the responsibility to take the necessary steps to provide care for the patient. If a malocclusion is diagnosed, he/she can consult an orthodontist and in some simple cases do the treatment him/herself under the supervision of the orthodontist. However, in most cases, the patient must be referred to a specialist for the best possible outcome, as children and teenagers with their parents currently demand a high extent of qualified orthodontic care. In other care systems or countries, it is normal that the patient and parents take the initiative to consult an orthodontist.

An increasing number of adults are seeking orthodontic correction of untreated malocclusions, irregularity of teeth, and late-developed crowding of teeth, as well as relapses of previous orthodontic treatment. The reason expressed by almost all of them is a desire for aesthetic improvement of dentofacial anomalies that, in many subjects, may cause psychosocial problems. One factor that should be stressed in relation to the demand for orthodontic treatment is the general social progress with emphasis on individual appearance and aesthetics. It is well known that treatment of severe malocclusions or dental anomalies positively affects a person's self esteem and psychological well-being, and for that reason, even treatment of minor deviations is justifiable in some sensitive individuals.

Consultations are also sought by dentists to align teeth and improve the position of the remaining teeth to facilitate prosthetic restorations, for realignment of teeth caused by pathological tooth migration, or in surgical treatment of severe malocclusions. This indicates that orthodontic treatment in those individuals is aimed at occlusal stability and chewing comfort. A comprehensive analysis and treatment plan must be based on a discussion between the orthodontist and the dentist who is responsible for the periodontal, prosthodontic or surgical procedures. Both have to come to an agreement about the optimal goal for the patient, including financial considerations. A schedule including the various steps of the treatment is presented to the patient, who will be informed in detail about the time of each step in the total procedure. The patient will be instructed to follow an oral hygiene programme to avoid possible dental and gingival damage during the orthodontic treatment, and a strongly motivated adult patient will cooperate excellently. Not until these steps have been taken, can the treatment start.

Demographic considerations demonstrate that the median age of the population will increase. Thus, the orthodontist should develop the skills necessary to manage the increasing number of interdisciplinary adult orthodontic patients, not only from an orthodontic horizon but also from other perspectives, for example development of dental material.

Special centres for the treatment of children with cleft-lip-palate defects and craniofacial syndromes are established in most countries. Different specialists are involved, functioning as a multidisciplinary team. The orthodontist's role in the cleft palate team requires close collaboration with the other team members, in particular, the plastic surgeon, oral surgeon and the speech pathologist.

The rationale of timing and sequencing orthodontic treatment has been discussed according to four periods of development: neonatal or infant maxillary orthopaedics,

orthodontic considerations in the primary dentition, in the mixed dentition to include pre-surgical considerations before an alveolar bone grafting, and a final treatment of the permanent dentition with orthodontics alone or combined with orthognathic surgery. The ultimate outcome for team-based care of these patients is to have a fully rehabilitated individual who is satisfied with the treatment outcomes in terms of speech, facial and dental aesthetics, occlusal stability and function. The patient shall continue to receive conventional dental and medical care similar to any other adult to maintain optimal oral health.

Conclusions

Essential orthodontics implies a knowledge of classification of malocclusions and dental anomalies and knowledge of craniofacial growth and development, and to be able to examine and communicate with the prospective orthodontic patient regarding the diversity of the orthodontic panorama.

CHAPTER 2
Classification of malocclusions

Lars Bondemark

Key topics

- Normal occlusion and malocclusions
- Discrepancies between the jaws – sagittal, vertical and transversal malocclusions
- Anomalies within the jaws – crowding, spacing, variations in number and malpositions of teeth
- Frequency of malocclusions
- Orthodontic treatment need

Learning objectives

- To be able to distinguish between normal occlusion and malocclusions
- To be able to classify malocclusions between and within the jaws, as well as categorise different malpositions of teeth
- To understand different malocclusions and their frequencies
- To understand what orthodontic treatment need means and what type of malocclusions should or should not be treated

Essential Orthodontics, First Edition. Birgit Thilander, Krister Bjerklin and Lars Bondemark.
© 2018 John Wiley & Sons Ltd. Published 2018 by John Wiley & Sons Ltd.

Normal occlusion and malocclusion

Normal, or ideal, occlusion is a concept constructed by the orthodontic profession. More than 100 years ago, Edward H. Angle introduced the first clear and simple definition of normal occlusion:

> The upper first molars are the key to occlusion and the upper and lower molars should be related so that the mesiobuccal cusp of the upper molar occludes in the buccal grove of the lower molar. If the teeth are arranged on a smoothly curving line of occlusion and this molar relationship exists, then normal occlusion would result (Angle, 1900).

The opposite condition is malocclusion, which was once defined as:

> The nature of malocclusion, not a disease, but rather a variation from accepted societal norm that can lead to functional difficulties or concerns about dento-facial appearance for a patient (Brook and Shaw, 1989).

Deviation from normal or ideal occlusion does not necessarily mean that the malocclusion needs to be treated. Assessment of treatment requirement is based on an evaluation of the risk, short or long term, for disturbances in oral health, function, aesthetics or patient satisfaction.

Usually, an occlusion or malocclusion is classified according to terms of discrepancies between the jaws, for example sagittal (anterior-posterior), vertical and transversal relationships including functional abnormalities between the maxillary and mandibular dental arches. In addition, anomalies within the jaws, for example crowding and spacing, variations in number of teeth and malpositions of teeth are considered. Some malocclusions, for example increased overjet, crowding and spacing. may be classified by range in millimetres. This implies that normal occlusions may have minor variations within a range and so is not a fixed condition. Furthermore, in sagittal, vertical and transversal discrepancies, skeletal deviations can be involved, combining both dental and skeletal discrepancies.

Discrepancies between the jaws

Sagittal plane

In the sagittal classification, the basis for assessment is the intermaxillary positions of the first molars. There exist three characteristics: normal, postnormal (Angle Class II) and prenormal (Angle Class III) occlusion.

Normal occlusion

In a normal sagittal occlusion, also called Angle Class I, the mesio-buccal cusp of the maxillary first molar occludes with the mesio-buccal groove of the mandibular first molar (Figure 2.1). The maxillary canine cusp tip occludes between the mandibular canine and first premolar (Figure 2.1). In principle, deviations of up to half a cusp width in a mesial or distal direction are considered a normal occlusion. The overjet in normal occlusions is usually between 2 and 5 mm. Sometimes the first molars have migrated because of early extraction of primary teeth due to, for example, caries. In such cases, the position of first molars prior to migration has to be estimated, and the

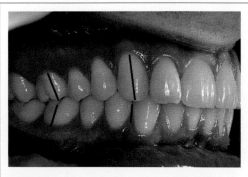

Figure 2.1 Angle Class I occlusion (normal occlusion).

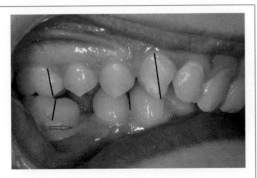

Figure 2.2 Normal sagittal molar relation because of mesial movement of the mandibular molar (arrow). However, the intermaxillary canine relationship indicates a Class II malocclusion, and thus this case shows a Class II malocclusion.

intermaxillary canine position can provide guidance (Figure 2.2).

Angle Class II occlusion

In an Angle Class II, or postnormal, occlusion, the mandibular first molar has a posterior position compared with normal occlusion, i.e. behind the normal position or in a distal relationship (Figure 2.3). In about 90% of the Angle Class II occlusions, the maxillary incisors are proclined, i.e. Angle Class II division 1 (Figure 2.4a), while approximately 10% show retroclined maxillary central incisors, i.e. Angle Class II division 2 (Figure 2.4b). In an Angle Class II division 1 occlusion, the overjet is often

enlarged, and if the overjet is over 6 mm, it is counted as great, and anything above 9 mm is considered extreme.

Angle Class III occlusion

Angle Class III, or prenormal, occlusion is evident when the mandibular first molar is in a prenormal position compared to the normal occlusion, i.e. in front of the normal position, or in a mesial relationship (Figure 2.5). In cases of Angle Class III occlusion, the overjet is often reversed (<0 mm), implying an anterior crossbite.

Vertical plane

Two possibilities are evident: open bite or deep bite.

Open bite

In open bite, there is no intermaxillary tooth contact, either in the front or laterally from the dental arch (Figure 2.6). To qualify as open bite, the overbite is reversed (<0 mm), and the teeth are assumed to be fully erupted.

Deep bite

Deep bite is defined as an excessive vertical overlap of the incisors, i.e. vertically, where more than two-thirds of the buccal surfaces of the mandibular incisors are covered by the maxillary incisors (Figure 2.7). Most often, the reason for deep bite is an over-eruption of the incisors or an anterior rotation of the mandible. A deep bite occasionally manifests with contact between the edges of the mandibular incisors and the palatal mucosa behind the maxillary incisors (Figure 2.8). In such cases, the contact between incisors and the mucosa may cause tissue ulceration. Therefore, the classification of deep bite includes evaluating whether contact exists between incisors and palatal mucosa and whether ulcerations occur.

Transversal plane

Transversal plane discrepancies relate to the width of the maxilla and/or mandible, and

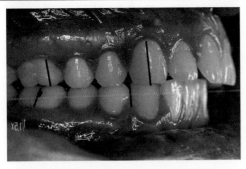

Figure 2.3 Angle Class II malocclusion (postnormal occlusion).

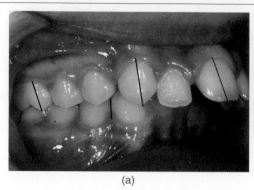
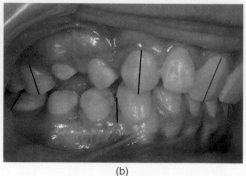

(a)   (b)

Figure 2.4 Angle Class II division 1 malocclusion (a) with proclined maxillary incisors (red line in a), and Angle Class II division 2 malocclusion (b) with retroclined maxillary central incisors (purple line in b).

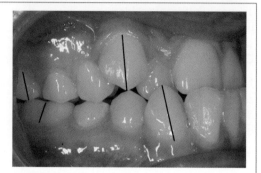

Figure 2.5 Angle Class III malocclusion (prenormal occlusion).

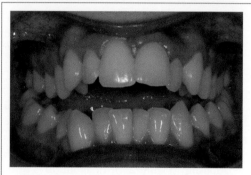

Figure 2.6 Open bite in the front between the jaws.

either posterior crossbite or scissors bite can be registered.

Posterior crossbite

In a posterior crossbite, the buccal cusps of the maxillary premolars and/or molars occlude lingually to the buccal cusps of the mandibular premolars and/or molars. The posterior crossbite can be either unilateral or bilateral. Unilateral crossbites of dento-alveolar origin are caused by palatal tipping of the maxillary premolars and molars, and is most often accompanied with a forced guidance of the mandible, thus deviating the midline of the mandible to the crossbite side (Figure 2.9) (Thilander and Myrberg, 1973). The force guidance has to be assessed or diagnosed in a clinical investigation.

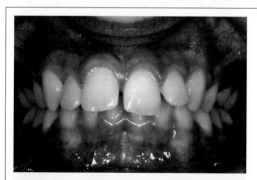

Figure 2.7 Deep bite.

A bilateral crossbite (Figure 2.10) is often caused by a transversal skeletal constriction of the maxilla and without a forced guidance of the mandible.

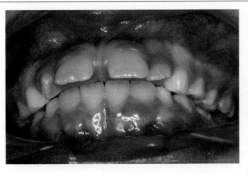

Figure 2.8 A deep bite with contact between the edges of the mandibular incisors and the palatal mucosa behind the maxillary incisors.

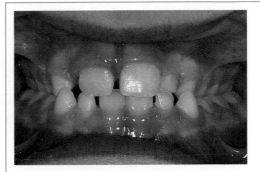

Figure 2.10 Bilateral crossbite.

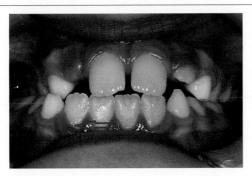

Figure 2.9 Unilateral crossbite on the right side of the individual, and there has been a forced guidance of the mandible, deviating the midline to the crossbite side (arrow).

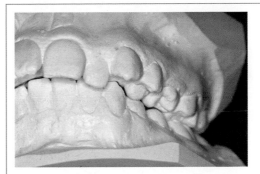

Figure 2.11 A scissors bite of maxillary left first and second premolar.

Scissors bite

In a scissors bite situation, one or more premolars or molars in the maxilla occlude with their lingual cusps buccal to the mandibular buccal cusps of the premolars and/or molars (Figure 2.11). Scissors bite may occur unilaterally or bilaterally and be associated with forced guidance of the mandible, but forced guidance is more infrequent than in posterior crossbites. Bilateral scissors bite is occasionally referred to as the Brodi syndrome.

Functional disturbances

When the bite is closing, and if the mandible is guided by an early intermaxillary abnormal contact, the mandible can either move laterally or in a forwards direction. When the mandible is guided laterally, a posterior crossbite is established (Figure 2.9), while if the mandible is forced forwards, an anterior crossbite will be created (Figure 2.12).

Anomalies within the jaws

Usually, the spatial conditions in the dental arches are determined by tooth size and the volume of the alveolar process. When the alveolar process of the jaw is undersized and, thereby, does not have enough space for the roots of the teeth, the occurring disproportion is called a small apical base that often results in proclined incisors and crowding (Figure 2.13). The opposite is a large apical base (Figure 2.14), which means that the alveolar process of the jaw is

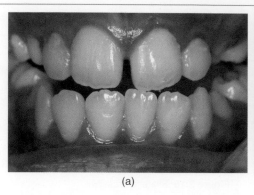
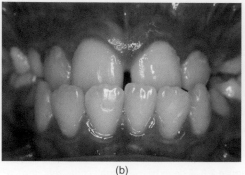

(a) (b)

Figure 2.12 Establishment of an anterior crossbite with functional shift. In a centric relationship, there is an edge-to-edge contact between maxillary and mandibular incisors (a). When the bite is closing, the mandible is guided in a forward/anterior direction and an anterior crossbite is created (b).

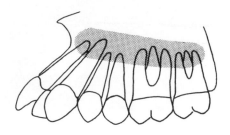

Figure 2.13 Undersized alveolar process, resulting in a small apical base with proclined incisors. The shaded area visualizes the small apical base.

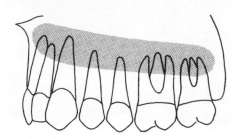

Figure 2.14 Large apical base resulting in vertical position of the maxillary incisors. The shaded area visualizes the large apical base.

oversized, resulting in vertical positions of the teeth and spacing (Lundström, 1923).

Crowding of teeth

Crowding is one of the most frequent malocclusions. A disparity of tooth size and the volume of the alveolar ridge will result in crowding with either lingually or buccally displaced teeth or rotations of teeth (Figure 2.15). Minor crowding of teeth is considered a normal condition; particularly, minor crowding in the mandibular incisor region is found in almost all individuals.

Spacing of teeth

Spacing is not as common as crowding, but spacing is frequently associated with small tooth size

in an otherwise normal or large alveolar ridge or dental arch. Spacing can also exist temporarily between the mixed and permanent dentition stages. An example of this is the median diastema in the mixed dentition (Figure 2.16). The diastema usually disappears when the lateral incisors and canines have fully erupted. If the diastema has not reduced or disappeared, it may be caused by pronounced frenula that can keep the central incisors away from each other with its inherent tissue forces (Figure 2.17).

Variations in number of teeth

Agenesis

Congenital absence of one or more teeth – agenesis, or hypodontia – is relatively common in the permanent dentition (Figure 2.18). It

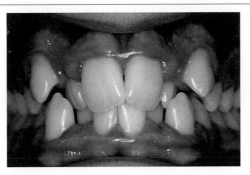

Figure 2.15 Crowding of teeth in the maxillary and mandibular anterior regions.

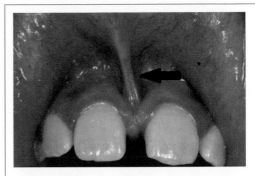

Figure 2.17 A pronounced frenula (arrow) that keeps the central incisors away from each other, resulting in a large median diastema.

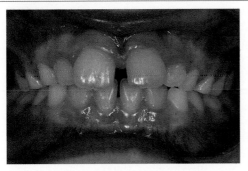

Figure 2.16 Spacing between the maxillary central incisors, i.e. a median diastema.

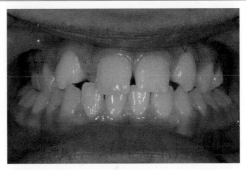

Figure 2.18 Congenital absence, agenesis, of a maxillary left lateral incisor. The left canine is now in the position of the lateral incisor (arrow).

can be noted that usually the most distal tooth in each dental anatomy group will increasingly become affected by agenesis. Consequently, the lateral incisor, second premolar and third molar have the highest prevalence of agenesis. Agenesis may also be associated with reduction in size of the rest of teeth. Agenesis of six or more teeth is termed oligodontia and if all teeth are absent, the condition is named anodontia. Oligodontia, especially anodontia, is very rare and linked to the syndrome ectodermal dysplasia.

In the primary dentition, agenesis is rarely found, but if it occurs, 70 to 80% of those will also have agenesis in the permanent dentition.

Supernumerary

The prevalence of supernumerary teeth or hyperodontia is low, and if it occurs it is often an extra tooth in the maxillary incisor region,

i.e. a mesiodens (Figure 2.19). Even more rarely, a supernumerary premolar or molar can be found.

Overall, variations in the number of teeth are recommended to be diagnosed in the mixed dentition, and for that purpose a panoramic radiograph is a good tool and for mesiodens, apical intra oral radiographs.

Malpositions of teeth

During the establishment of the dentition, and particularly in the mixed dentition stage, ectopic eruption (disturbed eruption direction) of maxillary molars and maxillary canines can be found. In cases with ectopic erupted maxillary first molars, the molar has resorbed the distal part of the second primary molar during the

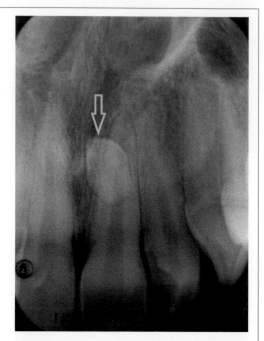

Figure 2.19 A supernumerary tooth in the maxillary incisor region, i.e. a mesiodens (arrow).

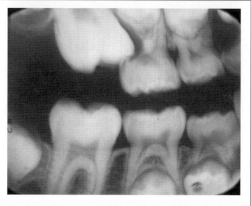

Figure 2.20 An ectopic erupted maxillary first permanent molar, and the molar has resorbed the distal part of the second primary molar.

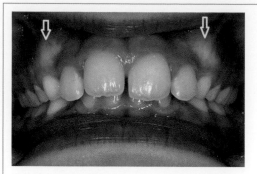

Figure 2.21 Bilaterally, the arrows point at the bumps buccally above the primary canines, indicating bilateral normal erupting canines.

eruption and the molar eruption has stopped (Figure 2.20). However, over 50% of ectopic molars will spontaneously free themselves in time from the primary molar and erupt (Bjerklin and Kurol, 1981).

To evaluate the eruption direction of the maxillary canine, it is advisable in the mixed dentition stage at 9 to 10 years of age, to palpate the maxillary alveolar ridge buccally above the primary canine. Normally, the canine can be palpated as a clear 'bump' on the alveolar ridge (Figure 2.21). If not palpable, it is desirable to take radiographs to evaluate the eruption of the canine (Figure 2.22).

It can also be recognised that individuals that have an ectopic erupted molar run a 50% higher risk of later developing an impacted canine (Bjerklin *et al.*, 1992).

Sometimes infraocclusion, a tooth or teeth which are below the occlusal plane of adjacent teeth, can be found in primary molars in the mixed dentition stage (Figure 2.23). The cause is ankylosis, which is an abnormal union or fusion that may occur between teeth and surrounding bone. Studies have shown that the infraoccluded primary molar will spontaneously exfoliate when the permanent successor erupts. Finally, a very rare condition is transposition, i.e. when an interchange of position of two permanent teeth exists (Figure 2.24).

Frequency of malocclusions

When describing how often a condition occurs or how many individuals belong to a particular category, the correct terminology is relative frequency. On the other hand, when describing the number of individuals in a population at a given time who have a certain disease, the term 'prevalence' is used. Since malocclusions are to be considered as variations from an accepted societal

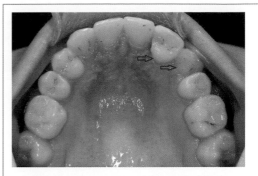

Figure 2.24 Transposition of the first maxillary premolar and canine. The premolar is mesially to the canine (arrows).

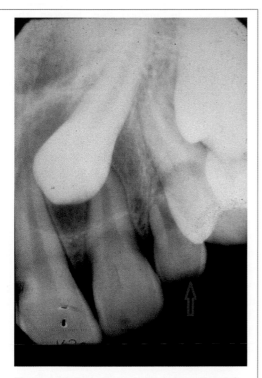

Figure 2.22 An ectopic positioned maxillary left canine. The position of the canine crown is far mesial than normal, and the primary canine is persisting (arrow).

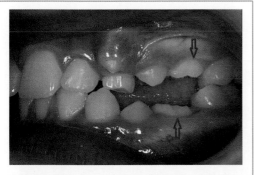

Figure 2.23 Infra occlusion of the primary maxillary and mandibular second molars (arrows).

norm rather than a disease, it is more accurate to use the term 'relative frequency' when describing how often malocclusions occur.

During dentofacial growth, and through the development from the primary to permanent dentition, malocclusions frequently exist.

When the frequency of malocclusions need be evaluated, there are different methods for classification:

a. the total frequency can be registered, i.e. a judgement as to whether any malocclusion exists or not;
b. typological classification, usually the Angle classification supplemented by further classes;
c. single traits of malocclusions based of an analysis of individual morphological variables, comprising metric and qualitative indices developed by Björk *et al.* (1964); and finally;
d. determining the individual malocclusion index, but these indices are more designed for evaluating the need for orthodontic treatment instead of the relative frequency of malocclusions.

Several studies have been conducted to evaluate the relative frequency of malocclusions, and the frequency of malocclusions is reported with a wide range of between 39 and 93% (Myllarniemi, 1970; Helm, 1970; Thilander and Myrberg, 1973; Lew *et al.*, 1993; Tschill *et al.*, 1997, Johannsdottir *et al.*, 1997; Thilander *et al.*, 2001; Dimberg *et al.*, 2015a). The range in relative frequency may reflect different methods and lack of conformity of methods of registration. However, it may also reflect variations in the size or composition of the population with respect to ethnicity and age, as well as whether orthodontic treatment has been carried out within the population, thereby reducing diverse malocclusions.

Table 2.1 A compilation of average frequency figures of the most common malocclusions occurring between mixed and permanent dentition.

Malocclusion	Frequency
Class II	14–18%
Class III	3–4%
Deep bite	8–11%
Open bite	4–5%
Posterior crossbite	8–12%
Scissors bite	1–2%
Crowding	25%
Spacing	9%
Agenesis (excluding 3rd molars)	6–8%
Supernumerary teeth	1%
Impacted maxillary canine	2–3%
Ectopic erupted first maxillary molar	4%
Infraoccluded primary molars	10–12%

Considering differences between ethnic groups, Class II malocclusions are much more frequent than Class III malocclusions in northern European populations, whereas in Asian populations, Class III malocclusions are more frequent than Class II malocclusions. Furthermore, anterior open bite is more frequent in African than in European populations.

Changes in malocclusion between the primary and permanent dentition have been shown, but the direction of the changes is difficult to predict (Foster and Grundy, 1986; Leighton and Feasby, 1988). Subsequently, self-correction of malocclusions has been reported for posterior crossbite and anterior open bites. A longitudinal study (Dimberg *et al.*, 2015a) revealed that at 3 years of age the relative frequency of malocclusion was 70%. At this age, anterior open bite predominated (50%), followed by increased overjet (23%) and posterior crossbite (19%). At 7 years of age, self-correction had occurred in all types of malocclusions, but new malocclusions had also developed. The amount of self-correction was higher than the development of new malocclusions, resulting in a total malocclusion frequency of 58%. Finally, at 11.5 years of age, the frequency of malocclusions was again at the same level as at the age of 3 (70%), but at this point the most frequent malocclusions are crowding followed by increased or excessive overjet and deep bite. In Table 2.1, some guidance figures are presented regarding the frequency levels for different malocclusions. Observe that combinations of malocclusions may occur, for example, an individual can simultaneously have a Class II malocclusion, deep bite and spacing (Figure 2.25).

It should be pointed out that when the relative frequency of malocclusions are evaluated,

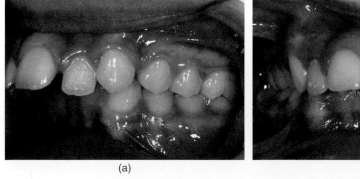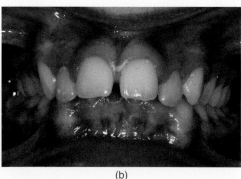

(a)	(b)

Figure 2.25 An individual showing multiple malocclusions, in this case Angle Class II division 1 malocclusion (a), together with deep bite and spacing (b).

well-defined populations with a sufficiently high amount of individuals must be obtained, and well-defined methods with strict criteria for registration of malocclusions should be used. Moreover, children and adolescents of different ages and without previous orthodontic treatment should be included. In addition, malocclusion is a clear appearance of morphological variations related to the development of the dentition instead of chronological age. Consequently, when the frequency of malocclusions shall be determined, it is more appropriate to relate the frequency to different stages of dental development rather than to different age groups.

Orthodontic treatment needs

A high frequency of malocclusions in a population does not necessarily imply that all individuals with malocclusions need orthodontic treatment. Assessment of treatment needs shall be based on an evaluation of the risk, in the short or long term, for disturbances in oral health, function, aesthetics or patient dissatisfaction. It is well-known that excessive overjet with incomplete lip closure, crowded incisors and large diastema between incisors (malocclusions in the aesthetic zone), have a negative impact on self-perceived oral health-related quality of life (Dimberg *et al.*, 2015a). Furthermore, subjects with Class II malocclusion and pre-treatment signs of temporomandibular disorders (TMD) of muscular origin benefit functionally from orthodontic treatment (Henrikson, 1999), and patients with severe dentofacial deformities, corrected by orthodontic treatment in conjunction with orthognathic surgery, have a positive treatment outcome in respect of TMD pain (Abrahamsson *et al.*, 2013).

One way to classify the orthodontic treatment need is to take *a careful selection of patients and in this context to use orthodontic-treatment-need indices.* Many different indices have been used, and the most common are the *Index of Orthodontic Treatment Need Dental Health Component* and *Index of Orthodontic Treatment Need Aesthetic Component* (IOTN-

DHC/IOTN-AC, Brook and Shaw, 1989), the *Index of Complexity Outcome and Need* (ICON, Daniels and Richmond, 2000), the *Dental Aesthetic Index* (DAI, Cons *et al.*, 1986), the *Index of Swedish National Board of Health* (Swe NBH, 1967) and the *Index of Norwegian Health Service* (Nor HS, 1986). These indices usually have four or five categories of orthodontic treatment needs, ranging from severe or very great to little or no need. Although several indices have been developed, to date none is considered sufficiently validated. Furthermore, a major drawback is that the patient's perspective is not properly considered (SBU, 2005). Nevertheless, these indices are currently the best tools available.

Several studies have been assessed to evaluate the orthodontic treatment needs (Thilander and Myrberg, 1973; Helm *et al.*, 1975; Heikinheimo, 1978; Rölling, 1978; Wheeler *et al.*, 1994; Perillo *et al.*, 2010; Dimberg *et al.*, 2015b). The results from these studies indicate that 35 to 40% of individuals in each population have a justified orthodontic treatment need to meet the requirements for a functional and aesthetically acceptable occlusion.

Conclusions

Usually, occlusion or malocclusion is classified according to terms of sagittal (anterior-posterior), vertical and transversal relationships between the maxillary and mandibular dental arches. Moreover, functional abnormalities, variations in number of teeth, malpositions of teeth, crowding and spacing shall be considered.

Several studies have been conducted to evaluate the frequency of malocclusions, and a wide range, between 39 and 93%, is reported. Despite a high frequency of malocclusions in a population, this does not necessarily imply that all individuals with malocclusions need orthodontic treatment. Nevertheless, it can be concluded that 35 to 40% of individuals in a population have a justified orthodontic treatment need to meet the requirements for a functional and aesthetically acceptable occlusion.

REFERENCES

Abrahamsson, C., Henrikson, T., Nilner, M. *et al.* (2013) TMD before and after correction of dentofacial deformities by orthodontic and orthognathic treatment. Int J Oral Maxillofac Surg 42: 752–758.

Angle, E.H. (1900) Treatment of malocclusion of the teeth and fractures of the maxillae. In: *Angle's System*, 6th edition. Philadelphia: SS White Dental Mfg. Co.

Bjerklin, K. and Kurol, J. (1981) Prevalence of ectopic eruption of the maxillary first permanent molar. Swed Dent J 5: 29–34.

Bjerklin, K., Kurol. J. and Valentin, J. (1992) Ectopic eruption of maxillary first permanent molars and association with other tooth and developmental disturbances. Eur J Orthod 14: 369–375.

Björk, A., Krebs, A. and Solow, B. (1964) A method of epidemiological registration of malocclusion. Acta Odont Scand 22: 27–41.

Brook, P.H. and, Shaw, W.C. (1989) The development of an index of orthodontic treatment priority. Eur J Orthod 11: 309–320.

Cons, N.C., Jenny, J. and Kohaut, F.J. (1986) *DAI: Dental Aesthetic Index*. College of Dentistry, University of Iowa, Iowa City.

Daniels, C. and Richmond, S. (2000) The development of the Index of Complexity, Outcome and Need (ICON). J Orthod 27: 149–162.

Dimberg, L., Lennartsson, B., Arnrup, K. *et al.* (2015a) Prevalence and change of malocclusions from primary to early permanent dentition: a longitudinal study. Angle Orthod 85: 728–734.

Dimberg, L., Arnrup, K. and Bondemark, L. (2015b) The impact of malocclusion on the quality of life among children and adolescents: a systematic review of quantitative studies. Eur J Orthod 37: 238–247.

Foster, T.D. and Grundy, M.C. (1986) Occlusal changes from primary to permanent dentitions. Br J Orthod 13: 187–193.

Heikinheimo, K. (1978) Need of orthodontic treatment in 7-year-old Finnish children. Community Dent Oral Epidemiol 6: 129–134.

Helm, S. (1970) Prevalence of malocclusion in relation to development of the dentition. An epidemiological study of Danish school children. Acta Odontol Scand Suppl No. 58.

Helm, S., Kreiborg, S., Barlebo, J. *et al.* (1975) Estimates of orthodontic treatment need in Danish schoolchildren. Community Dent Oral Epidemiol 3: 136–142.

Henrikson, T. (1999) Temporomandibular disorders and mandibular function in relation to Class II malocclusion and orthodontic treatment. A controlled, prospective and longitudinal study. Swed Dent J Suppl 134: 1–144 (Thesis).

Johannsdottir, B., Wisth, P.J. and Magnusson, T.E. (1997) Prevalence of malocclusion in 6-year-old Icelandic children. Acta Odontol Scand 55: 398–402.

Leighton, B.C. and Feasby, W.H. (1988) Factors influencing the development of molar occlusion: a longitudinal study. Br J Orthod 15: 99–103.

Lew, K.K., Foong, W.C. and Loh, E. (1993) Malocclusion prevalence in an ethnic Chinese population. Aust Dent J 38: 442–449.

Lundström, A. (1923) Malocclusions of the teeth regarded as a problem in connection with the apical base. Int J Orthod 11.

Myllarniemi, S. (1970) Malocclusion in Finnish rural children – An epidemiological study of different stages of dental development. Suom Hammaslaak Toim 66: 219–264.

Norwegain Health Service Nor HS (1986) Folketrygdens finansiering av tannhelsearbeid. Universitetsforlaget, Oslo NOU, 25.

Perillo, L., Masucci, C., Ferro, F. *et al.* (2010) Prevalence of orthodontic treatment need in southern Italian schoolchildren. Eur J Orthod 32: 49–53.

Rölling, S. (1978) Orthodontic examination of 2,301 Danish children aged 9–10 years in a community dental service. Community Dent Oral Epidemiol 6: 146–150.

SBU – Swedish Council on Technology Assessment in Health Care (2005) Malocclusions and orthodontic treatment in a health perspective: a systematic review of literature. SBU report 176, Stockholm.

Swedish National Board of Health Swe NBH. (1967) Kungliga Medicinalstyrelsens circular, Stockholm, M.F. No. 71.

Tschill, P., Bacon, W. and Sonko, A. (1997) Malocclusion in the deciduous dentition of Caucasian children. Eur J Orthod 19: 361–367.

Thilander, B. and Myrberg, N. (1973) The prevalence of malocclusion in Swedish schoolchildren. Scand J Dent Res 81: 12–21.

Thilander, B., Pena, L., Infante, C. *et al.* (2001) Prevalence of malocclusion and orthodontic treatment need in children and adolescents in Bogota, Colombia. An epidemiological study related to different stages of dental development. Eur J Orthod 23: 153–167.

Wheeler, T.T., McGorray, S.P., Yurkiewicz, L. *et al.* (1994) Orthodontic treatment demand and need in third and fourth grade schoolchildren. Am J Orthod Dentofacial Orthop 106: 22–33.

CHAPTER 3
Craniofacial growth and development

Birgit Thilander

Key topics

- Developmental periods and growth in height (stature)
- Standards of growth and development
- Prenatal development
- Postnatal growth and development of the craniofacial complex
- Growth of the nasomaxillary complex
- Growth of the mandible
- Development of the dentoalveolar complex
- Eruption of teeth and development of the dental arches and occlusion
- Development of the dental arches and occlusion

Learning objectives

- To understand the definitions and standards of growth
- To understand prenatal development
- To understand postnatal growth and development of the craniofacial complex
- To understand the development of the dentoalveolar complex
- To understand and have knowledge of the eruption mechanisms of the teeth

Essential Orthodontics, First Edition. Birgit Thilander, Krister Bjerklin and Lars Bondemark.
© 2018 John Wiley & Sons Ltd. Published 2018 by John Wiley & Sons Ltd.

Introduction

The fully developed cranium represents the sum of its separate parts, in which growth is highly differentiated and occurs at different rates and in different directions, and is a very complex concept. Knowledge of the normal process provides a basis for correct diagnosis of a malocclusion and is consequently a prerequisite for optimal orthodontic treatment in the individual case. Changes in the soft tissue profile with age follow the growth in the underlying hard tissues and are of importance in treatment planning, due to aesthetics.

The development and growth of the skull comprise phenomena falling within the scope of several disciplines and occurring at several levels. No specific method can therefore be assigned to the study of craniofacial growth. However, both experimental and clinical methods have been applied. Twin studies have been used to elucidate the importance of heredity and environmental factors. Biometric methods (longitudinal, semi-longitudinal or cross-sectional types) are suited for dimensional changes during growth. X-ray cephalometry is an often-used method for longitudinal follow-ups, and our information on human craniofacial growth is to a large extent based on that technique. The most commonly-used methods are experiments on laboratory animals to explain how cranial growth is regulated by studying specific events at the cell and tissue level by using histological, biochemical and histochemical techniques. In recent years, studies at the molecular level have additionally increased our knowledge of bone biology. The outcome from all these methods forms the basis for modern knowledge of craniofacial growth, which can be divided into four components:

1 growth mechanism (how new bone is formed);
2 growth pattern (change in size and shape of the bone);
3 growth rate (speed at which the bone is formed); and
4 the regulation mechanism, which initiates and directs those three processes.

Definitions of general growth

Growth, in a biological sense, is usually defined as an increase in size or weight of a tissue, an organ or an individual, and can be described quantitatively by diagrams or curves. The change in growth intensity over time is obvious when expressed as a velocity or rate curve (Figure 3.1), as used to describe the pubertal growth spurt in adolescence. The growth rate differs markedly from one organ or tissue system, even showing periods of regression. Growth in a tissue is genetically controlled but is also influenced by other factors, for example race, sex, nutrition and state of health.

Growth is often used as a synonymous for development which, in a biological sense, is defined as any process of continuous changes, and is therefore a broader term involving both quantitative and qualitative changes. The term 'differentiation' is used to describe development from a homogenous entity to increased complexity and specialisation at the cellular and tissue level, which are prerequisites of

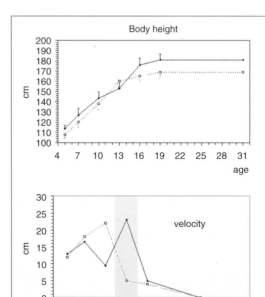

Figure 3.1 Mean growth in body height and velocity for Swedish boys and girls from 5 years of age to 31 years. Girls – dotted lines.

morpho-differentiation, i.e. the development in shape and size that determines the morphology of organs, systems and the whole body. Disturbance of this process may result in congenital defects.

The stage that the individual has reached in the process of development is usually described by the term 'maturation'. It is a very broad term, but usually refers to a specific organ or functional system, and is described in relation to specific features. Physical maturation may thus be described in terms of developmental age, which often does not coincide with chronological age. The great individual variation in growth due to genetic, social and nutritional factors makes developmental age a more suitable measure of development than chronological age.

Developmental periods and growth in height (stature)

Based on the average fluctuation in growth and maturation, the following developmental periods up to adulthood are generally recognized. Each of them is characterised by special growth and developmental features, but there are no sharp boundaries between them.

The prenatal stage is classified into ovum period (1st week), embryonic period (2nd–7th weeks) and foetal period (8th–40th weeks). The growth rate, largely determined by maternal factors, is low in the embryo. The foetus, however, has a high growth factor while undergoing morphological differentiation, especially during the 5th month. The weight gain per unit time, on the other hand, is greatest towards the end of the foetal period, and at birth the child will be about 50 to 52 cm long with a weight of round 3,500 g.

During the postnatal stage, the growth rate is related to the individual's genetic background, and is usually divided into the following four different periods:

1 *In the infantile period* – (1–12 months after birth) the rate of growth declines considerably as the effect of foetal growth fades. A simple rule of thumb is that the child's height at the age of 2 years is about a half of its final height in adulthood.

2 *The juvenile period* – (early childhood at the age of 1–6 years and late childhood at the age of 7–10 years) is characterized by relatively slow growth with a decline in rate towards a pre-puberty minimum, which in Scandinavia occurs at the age of about 10.5 years in girls and 11.5 years in boys. There are great variations, however, and the range for the pre-puberty minimum is held to be as much as 4 years. A pre-puberty growth acceleration even occurs between 6 and 8 years of age.

3 *The puberty* – (early adolescence) features a growth spurt with a peak height of velocity (PHV) at about 12.5 years in girls and about 14 years in boys. The individual variation in the rate and timing of this peak is again about 4 years for both sexes. Girls reach their peak earlier than boys. The growth rate declines after PHV at about the same speed as during the infantile period (Figure 3.1).

4 Growth gradually ceases during late adolescence and is generally completed by the age of 20 years, which is the point in time when growth in stature is less than 0.5 cm in 2 years and adulthood is reached.

Standards of growth and development

To estimate the individual growth and maturation, standards or criteria of normality are needed, to which individual deviations can be related. Standards of growth and development are normally given as mean values obtained in studies of representative groups from a population whose variation is assumed to lie within the normal range. Normal growth in a child should therefore be determined by the fact that it falls within the range of variation of the child's potential growth in its social environment.

The dentition as well as the jaws will show large variation in developmental level in a group of children, for example classmates, when related to chronological age, which provides only a rough estimate of developmental level. In order to judge deviations from a normal pattern, this variation has to be considered in orthodontic diagnosis and treatment planning. It is of the greatest importance to estimate the biological age of the child, which involves the following different types of developmental ages:

■ *Morphological age* – is a comparison of attained size (height and weight) to normative standards. There is a close correlation between the growth spurt in skeletal height (stature) and various facial dimensions, while it has been proposed that longitudinal recording of body height is a useful aid for the planning of orthodontic treatment. A factor of general interest is the secular trend in mean height in Scandinavian schoolchildren during the 20th century (Brundtland *et al.*, 1980).

■ *Skeletal age* – provides a record of the developmental age of the growing skeleton. Skeletal maturation follows a predetermined pattern, since some bones mature faster than others, and can be assessed by X-raying the hand and wrist. Maturity stages based on hand X-rays can be useful complements to body height measurements and lateral head X-rays.

■ *Dental age* – may also be used to describe physical maturity. While sexual age and skeletal age are closely related in normal growth, while dental and skeletal maturity show weak correlation. Several systems have been developed to estimate the dental age from radiographs (Demirjian and Godstein, 1976). The dental age is above all used in estimating the age of a child with unknown birth date and in forensic medicine.

■ *Dental stage* – is a term introduced by Björk *et al.* (1964). Instead of age, the children are grouped according to their tooth emergence status. Dental stages are very useful in clinical work, both in diagnosis and in treatment planning.

Prenatal development of the face and jaws

A good knowledge of prenatal development is necessary for a proper understanding of the postnatal growth and the pathogenesis of congenital facial malformations. The germ layers, which form the basis of the embryogenesis of the different organ systems, are:

1 *The endoderm* – gives rise to the epithelial lining in the posterior part of the oral cavity and the entire digestive system, from the root of the tongue downwards.

2 *The ectoderm* – gives rise to the skin and related structures (hair, nails and sweat glands), nervous system, nasal epithelium, the epithelial lining of the anterior part of the oral cavity, and the tooth enamel.

3 *The mesoderm* – gives rise to the mesenchyme (embryonic connective tissue), differentiating into connective tissue, skeleton and smooth muscles (except in the skin), blood and lymphatic tissues.

4 *The ectomesenchyme* – is often described as a fourth germ layer. It derives from the neural crest cells, a population of cells that arises at the boundary of the embryonic neural folds during formation of the neural tube. They separate from the ectoderm on the 21st to 22nd day, after which they undergo intensive migration sub-ectodermally. They give rise to a variety of structures in the facial region, including skeletal and dental tissues. As these migrating cells control normal growth along their paths, deviations from this development can occur at various times and stages in neural crest formation, differentiation and morphogenesis (Ten Cate, 1980).

In the early embryonic period, the germ disc becomes increasingly curved, especially in its cranial and caudal parts where head and tail are established (Figure 3.2). At the same time, a swelling arises at its cephalic part, marking the development of the anterior brain vesicle, the prosencephalon. In this way, the head gains its characteristic forward bend at the vertebral column flexure during the second month. The first external sign of the formation of the sense organs can now be seen in the form of epithelial lens and otic placodes. The head of the foetus develops rapidly from now on, and by the end of the embryonic period, it shows the external features of a human being. During the latter part of this period, a cartilaginous skeleton of the head, the chondrocranium, develops, followed

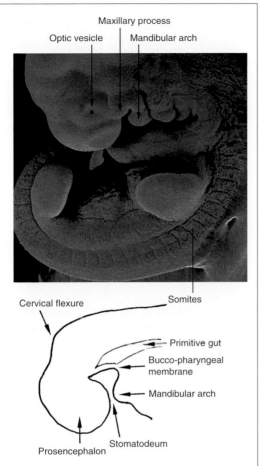

Maxillary process

Optic vesicle   Mandibular arch

Cervical flexure   Somites

Primitive gut

Bucco-pharyngeal membrane

Mandibular arch

Prosencephalon   Stomatodeum

Figure 3.2 At the top, the mesoderm on each side of the neural tube splits into segments (somites) in an embryo at 4 weeks. At the bottom is seen a mid-sagittal section with the primitive oral cavity.

by the first ossification centres in the face, the jaws and the cranial base.

Development of the face and jaws

The cephalic part of a 3-week embryo (3 mm) is dominated by the procencephalon. Above is a depression (stomatodeum) forming the primitive oral cavity (Figure 3.2). On each side of this depression, the branchial or pharyngeal arches start to develop, with bulges on the ecto-dermal surface and pouches on the endodermal surface. The primitive oral cavity will by this time be surrounded by the first branchial arch (the mandibular arch) and the small maxillary

processes developing bilaterally from its dorsal portions. The stomatodeum deepens further, but is still separated from the foregut by the bucco-pharyngeal membrane, which is made up of an outer ectodermal layer towards the stomatodeum and an inner endodermal layer towards the primitive gut. Disintegration of the membrane at the 28th day involves connection between the stomatodeum and the foregut is established. From this it is easy to under-stand while the epithelia of the oral and nasal cavities and tooth enamel are of ectodermal origin, while the pharyngeal epithelium is of endodermal origin.

The nasomaxillary complex takes shape as a consequence of continuing differentiation and growth of the ectomesenchyme via:

1 the medial and lateral nasal processes from the frontal process, which in turn develops from procencephalon; and
2 the two maxillary processes, developing as separate entities from the dorsal portions of the 1st branchial arch (Figure 3.3).

The medial process grows caudally to join the anteriorly and medially processes, resulting in an incomplete roof to the mouth (*the primary palate*). The medial nasal process forms the central part of the nose and the central part of the upper lip. The roof of the mouth thus is a horseshoe-shaped structure with its anterior part formed by the primary palate and its lateral boundaries by the maxillary processes. There remains considerable confusion regarding the mechanism of the formation of the primary palate, but evidently a small part is initially formed by an epithelial invagination, whereas the major part is formed by coalescence of the facial processes, apparently through epithelial fusion and ectomesenchymal penetration for consolidation (Ferguson, 1991). Clefts in the primary palate may thus result from failure at various stages of these processes. The 6th week is critical for these clefts (Figure 3.4).

During the 7th week, two tissue folds (palatal shelves), developing from the max-illary processes, grow in vertical–anterior directions on each side of the developing tongue (Figure 3.5a). About a week later they rise into a horizontal position above the tongue (Figure 3.5b). Fusion of the shelves

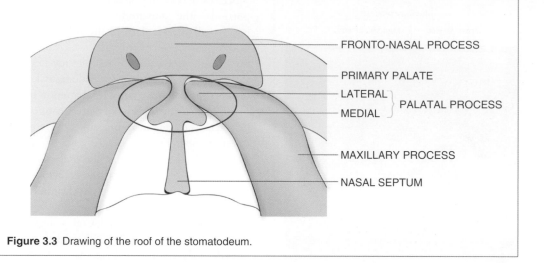

Figure 3.3 Drawing of the roof of the stomatodeum.

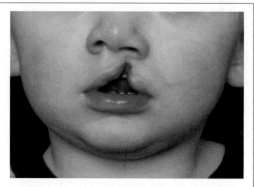

Figure 3.4 A child with a cleft lip.

proceeds in a posterior direction from the 8th to the 12th week (Figure 3.5c). Establishment of the secondary palate thus includes two determinative events: reorientation of the palatal shelves and their subsequent fusion in the midline. Failure in this synchronism involves defective closure and results in a cleft. Combined cleft lip and palate (CLP) may occur uni- or bilaterally (Figure 3.6).

The 1st branchial arch makes up the mandible during the embryonic period, with a cartilage rod (Meckel's cartilage) acting as the primary skeleton for the lower face. This cartilage later retrogresses, except dorsally, where it remains as a ligament and as a precursor to the auditory ossification of the ear. In the 6th

to 7th weeks, parts of the ossified mandibular corpus can be seen in the shape of thin bone plates in the area of the mental foramen and lateral to Meckel's cartilage. The ossified corpus and ramus of the mandible are formed by expansion anteriorly and posteriorly, and will remain as a paired structure throughout the foetal period.

Between the 10th and 12th weeks, the ectomesenchyme differentiates into a secondary cartilage in the condylar area, extending cranially and inferiorly towards the expanding mandibular body. The temporomandibular joint (TMJ) has in principle assumed its final form by the end of the 4th month. When compared with other synovial joints in the body, it is late in forming, which may be explained by its origin as a secondary cartilage, while the regulating mechanism of synovial joint development is of muscular origin.

Ossification of the craniofacial skeleton

The first sign of skeletal development is an increased density in the ectomesenchyme in the 2nd foetal month, which differentiates into a hyaline cartilage skeleton, the chondrocranium, mainly comprising the anterior part of the cranial base and the nasal capsule. Several ossification centres appear in these structures, from which the large part of the chondrocranium

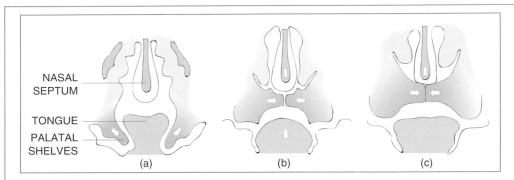

Figure 3.5 Drawings of different stages in development of the secondary palate, anterior section.

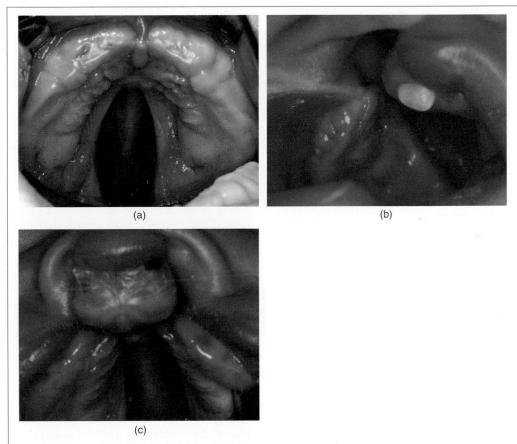

Figure 3.6 A palatal cleft (a), a unilateral CLP (b), a bilateral CLP (c).

is ossified during the foetal period. Remnants persist as cartilaginous joints, synchondroses. At the same time, several ossification centres develop in the facial region and, somewhat later, in the soft tissue membrane around the brain. These ossification centres rapidly expand to form the facial skeleton and vault of the cranium,

the desmocranium. When intramembraneously formed bones meet, sutures develop.

Facial muscles

The participation of the myotomes (differentiated from the somites) in the development of the muscles in the head region is a subject of controversy. Out of the total of 42 to 44 pairs of myotomes, only 4 (the occipital myotomes) are established in the cephalic region, and one of them regresses. The facial muscles are thought to develop from the ectomesenchyme of the pharyngeal arches and the differentiation to form the separate muscles is extremely complex, as it is characterised by an intense migration in many directions. The muscles of mastication develop from the 1st pharyngeal arch (innervated by the Vth cranial nerve), whereas the mimic muscles differentiate from the 2nd pharyngeal arch (innervated by the VII cranial nerve). Despite their migration, the separate muscles and nerves supplying them remain intimately associated throughout the developmental period. Neuromuscular activity in the orofacial muscles has been observed as early as during the 3rd foetal month.

The anterior part of the tongue develops from the mandibular arch and the posterior part of the second, third, and part of the fourth pharyngeal arches. Establishing the *tongue muscles* starts during the 7th week, but their origin is uncertain. Comparative anatomical studies and the innervation data indicate that the occipital myotomes participate in its ontogenesis. According to another theory, the muscles of the tongue develop directly from the mesenchyme and are not related to the myotomes. This would explain why so many nerves are involved in its innervation (V, VII, IX and XII cranial nerves).

Postnatal growth and development of the craniofacial complex

At the time of birth, the craniofacial skeleton has undergone almost half of its total growth and the head makes up about a quarter of the body height, whereas in adults it is about one-eighth of the body height. Although this reflects the early development of the final size of the head compared with the rest of the body, the remaining dimensional increase is not equal in all parts of the cranium. While the size of the cerebral cranium will increase by about 50%, the facial skeleton will grow

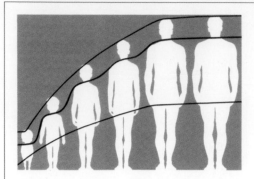

Figure 3.7 Diagram illustrating the proportions in body height at different ages. Note the relation between the head and the body at the different ages.

to more than twice the size (Figure 3.7). This difference in proportions is associated with the early development of the brain, whose growth is practically completed by the age of 4 years.

The facial skeleton increases in all dimensions, that of height being the greatest (~200%), that of depth somewhat smaller (~150%), and that of width the smallest (~75%). Facial width is one of the first three dimensions to reach normal size, and the facial skeleton therefore becomes steadily longer and narrower from birth to adulthood.

Ethnic differences in facial traits exist, and the dentofacial pattern will change during periods of active growth, as has been reported in many studies of cephalometric norms or standards for individuals of varying ethnic groups and ages. This can be illustrated by superimposed tracings from individuals with normal (ideal) occlusion, followed from 5 years up to 31 years of age (Thilander *et al.*, 2005) (Figure 3.8). As can be seen, facial pattern changes exist during the observation period, with growth acceleration between the 13 and 16 years recordings. Obvious changes are noted also in the period between 5 and 7 years of age as well as between 16 and 31 years, and changes in adults older than that have been reported (Bondevik, 2012). Thus, a sound knowledge of growth and development in 'normal' individuals are essential in diagnosing each malocclusion. Growth and development of the different parts in the dentofacial entity (cranial base, nasomaxillay

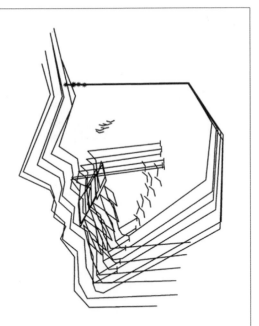

Figure 3.8 Superimposed tracings from individuals of 5 to 31 years of age and with normal occlusion.

complex, and mandible) form the basis for a detailed diagnosis (differential diagnosis) and the treatment planning in patients with any type of malocclusions.

Mechanism of bone growth

Bone grows by two fundamental physiologic processes; modelling and remodelling. Modelling is a surface-specific activity that shapes and changes the size and shape of the bone, while remodelling occurs in the bone tissues as reconstruction of bone by turnover of previous osseous tissue (Haversian system) and regulation at the molecular level. The process we are dealing with in facial morphogenesis is growth remodelling, i.e. both modelling and remodelling are included in this term.

Bone growth in the craniofacial complex is under genetic control and is influenced by epigenetic and environmental factors. Developmentally, bone formation occurs either by endochondral ossification with a cartilage model, or by a direct intramembranous formation. Although the starting processes are different, once formed, bones of both origins

are modelled and remodelled in the same way. The skeleton is a dynamic and complex mineralized connective tissue with high capacity to adapt to various mechanical and physiological requirements, in which osteoclastic bone resorption and osteoblastic bone formation are highly coordinated. The periosteum is of greatest significance in this process and hence for the change in size and shape of the bones (growth pattern).

The inner cambium layer of the periosteum provides the mesenchymal stem cells and osteoprogenitor cells, required for growth and development of the bone (Roberts *et al.*, 2015). Mesenchymal stem cells are recruited from the circulation, bone marrow or the periosteum to the site for new bone formation. The commitment of mesenchymal stem cells to osteoprogenitor cells and ultimately to differentiated osteoblasts is regulated by several factors, which are bound to specific receptors, for example bone morphogenetic proteins (BMPs), belonging to the transforming growth factor-ß (TGFß) family, and fibroblast growth factors (FGFs) (Capulli *et al.*, 2014). The fully differentiated osteoblast is characterized by alkaline phosphatase activity and production of proteins, for example collagen type I and more bone-specific non-collagenous proteins. Osteoblasts are seen either at the bone surface or within lacunae in the newly-formed matrix (Figure 3.9). They occur as active cuboidal cells or as inactive flat bone-lining cells (Figure 3.9).

The remodelling cycle starts with osteoclastic resorption and is subsequently followed by new bone formation at the same site, which occurs in coordinated functional basic multicellular units. The coupling mechanisms between osteoclastic bone resorption and the following bone formation are still not clear.

Osteoclasts are the only cells which can resorb mineralized tissues. New osteoclasts are actively recruited from hematopoietic stem cells of the monocyte-macrophage lineage when a resorption process is to start. The mononuclear osteoclast precursors fuse to form multinucleated cells with a short life span. Osteoclasts adhere tightly to the bone surface and form a sealing zone, in which they, via a specialized ruffled border of the cell membrane, release proteolytic enzymes

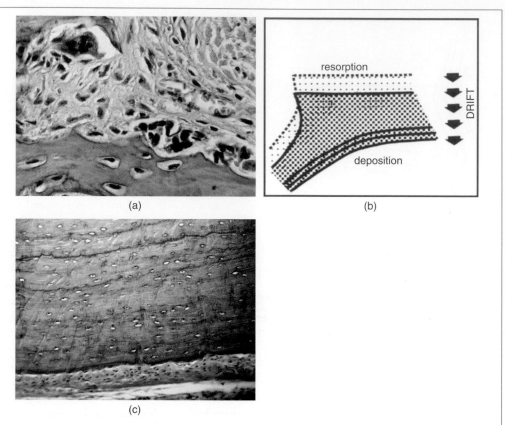

Figure 3.9 Illustration of relocation (drift) of the maxillary palate. Photomicrograph showing cuboidal cells at the resorption area (a), periosteal resorption on the nasal side and deposition on the oral side (b), and photomicrograph showing flat bone lining cells at the deposition area (c).

and hydrogen ions to degrade and resorb the organic and inorganic components of the bone. The activation of the osteoclast is crucially dependent on macrophage colony stimulating factor (M-CSF) and receptor activator of nuclear factor kappa-B ligand (RANKL), which is produced by osteoblasts in response to various factors, for example hormones, prostaglandins (PG) and pro-inflammatory cytokines. It has been recently discovered that osteocytes produce large amounts of RANKL and thus support osteoclastic bone resorption.

The osteocyte is the most common cell in the bone tissue, accounting for more than 90% of the cells, and estimated to have a 10 to 20 years life-span. Osteocytes are functionally connected to other cells via long cellular processes and gap junction channels. Many regulatory signals between osteocytes and other cells are mediated via gap junctional transport

of ions, small molecules and second messengers. Gap junction channels between two docking cells are formed by transmembrane connexion (Cx) proteins, of which Cx43 is the most widely expressed in osteoblasts and osteocytes (Civitelli, 2008). The Cx43 gap junction is crucial in normal osteoblast function, osteogenesis and craniofacial bone development (Lecanda *et al.*, 2000). Moreover, Cx43 and gap junction communication also seems to play an important role in signalling pathways linked to bone resorption. The osteoblast-osteocyte production of the osteoblast regulating cytokines RANKL and osteoprotegerin (OPG) is depending on functional Cx43 channels. Osteoclast precursors and mature osteoclasts are reported to express Cx43 proteins and direct signalling through gap junction channels is crucial for the development of osteoclasts and their bone resorbing activities (Ransjö *et al.*, 2003; Zappittelli *et al.*, 2014).

Bone growth implies a continuous replacement of matrix-producing cells via cell division in the cambium layer. Owing to their localization, both matrix-producing and proliferation cells are subject to mechanical influence. If the pressure exceeds a certain threshold level with reduced blood supply, the osteogenesis ceases and osteoclasts appear until biochemical equilibrium is restored. If, on the other hand, the periosteum is exposed to tension, it responds with bone apposition. The osteocytes are capable of sensing mechanical load and micro-damage in bone tissue and subsequently regulate the bone remodelling response. The continuous remodelling serves to maintain the shape and proportions of the bones throughout the growth period. As bone deposition occurs during the concomitant breakdown of opposing bone surfaces, the bone will migrate in relation to a fixed structure. In the orthodontic literature, this passive migration is known as relocation or drift, opposite to the more active movement, called translation or displacement. The periosteum continuous to function as an osteogenic zone throughout life, but its regenerative capacity is extremely high in the young child. Thus, the influence of the periosteum is of the greatest significance for the change in size and shape of the bones (growth pattern).

Growth of the cranial base

The cranial base constitutes the integrated part between the neurocranium and the visceral cranium. Its sagittal aspect, used as a reference plane in most cephalometric systems, is of special interest for the orthodontist. The cranial base consists of many different bones, and the timing of termination of growth at the various sites is of particular interest (Thilander and Ingervall, 1973; Melsen, 1974), illustrated in Figure 3.10. The anterior portion is stable by the age of 7 years, and its increase afterwards is due to bone apposition on the frontal and nasal bones, explicitly in males. The growth of the posterior part is not terminated until adolescence due to the spheno-occipital synchondrosis, the most important remnant of the prenatal cartilage.

The young human synchondrosis consists of a bipolar 'epiphyseal' plate with endochondral

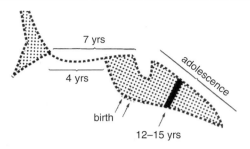

Figure 3.10 Drawing illustrating timing of the termination of growth in different parts of the cranial base.

ossification and its structural organization changes with age. The hyaline cartilage is partly replaced by fibrocartilage in its superior part during the first 1 to 2 years after birth. At that time the brain needs more space, being required for the child's balance when it starts walking. Thus, the occipital bone is pressed downwards, a movement that initiates a stress in the synchondrosis, which explains the translation into fibrocartilage. This area becomes narrower through ossification from both sides and is completely covered with bone by the age of 12 to 13 years in females and some years later in males.

The postnatal importance of the spheno-occipital synchondrosis, sometimes considered the driving force for cranial base growth, has been questioned. It is more likely that the cartilage plays a relatively greater role in the adjustment changes in the cranial base flexure than in its linear growth. The curvature of the cranial base is also correlated with head position, i.e. the relationship of the head to the cervical column. Functional requirements for breathing and swallowing can be fulfilled by variations of the head position and thus even may influence the craniofacial skeletal pattern (Solow and Tallgren, 1976; Huggare, 1995).

Growth of the nasomaxillary complex

A visceral cranium of a newborn will show the start of its postnatal growth and development. Development of the orbital cavities is practically complete at birth. The nasal cavity is located between the two orbits with its floor level with their bases. The alveolar process can only be discerned and the palate has a weak transversal curvature. The maxillary body is almost entirely filled with the developing teeth.

The nasomaxillary complex in its entirety is built up of several bones connected by sutures. The increase of each bony part is restricted to its surrounding periosteal surfaces. The nasal septum has also been considered of importance for the growth of the middle face. And the tooth-bearing units (alveolar processes) influence the growth in facial height. Therefore, the following growth areas are involved in the nasomaxillary complex: conversion of nasal septal cartilage, periosteal remodelling, sutural deposition and tooth eruption.

Nasal septal cartilage plays an important part in the prenatal and very early postnatal growth of the middle face. Opinions differ, however, considering its role later in life. According to Scott (1962), the septal cartilage occupies a unique location for pushing the whole maxilla forward. The opposing view, commonly termed 'the functional matrix' by Moss (1962), suggests that the nasal septal cartilage is a locus of secondary and compensatory growth. Many experimental studies have been performed to find evidence favouring those hypotheses. Experiments involving partial or total removal of the septum have given different result. Sarnat and Wexler (1968) found a significant decrease in growth of the nasal complex when such a procedure was carried out in young rabbits. Stenström and Thilander (1970), however, found only negligible changes in the dimension of the snout of growing guinea pigs after extirpation of the whole septum, i.e. results supporting Moss' theory. Pertinent literature on the role of the nasal septum in postnatal midfacial growth will conclude that its growth is secondary to and compensatory for a prior passive displacement of the midfacial bones, but it plays a biomechanical role in maintaining normal midfacial form.

Displacement growth is made possible by the craniofacial sutures, which have a dual function of permitting growth movement and uniting the bones of the cranium, while at the same time allowing slight movement in response to mechanical stress. Animal studies indicate that displacement of the bone due to growth can even regulate the development of the sutures (Persson, 1973). The sutures consist of fibrous tissue with osteogenic layers on both bone surfaces and so form an extension of the periosteal layer of the bone. Thereby they participate in the design of the bone by remodelling activity. The structure of the tissue, especially its fibrous component, varies and may be assumed to reflect the varying functional demands which endeavour to displace the bones in relation to one another. Tissue proliferation and bone deposition towards the suture borders thus have a space filling function and are secondary to separation of the bones from an external force. The fibrous component of the suture increases with age, and fibre bundles can be seen running transversally across the suture and further increasing the mechanical strength of the joint. When growth of the maxilla is finished, most sutures are ossified (Persson and Thilander, 1977; Persson et al., 1978).

Growth pattern of the maxilla

Depth The dimensional increase of the maxilla takes place in the posterior direction by bone deposition on the tuberosity and adjacent sutures, resulting in displacement of the two maxillary bodies. In relation to the cranial base, the maxillary growth occurs in an anterior–inferior direction, although there are great individual variations. The alveolar base is thereby elongated, creating space for posterior and late erupting teeth. The anterior surface of the maxilla, on the other hand, is fairly stable from a growth point of view and only exhibits a remodelling pattern.

In this displaced maxilla, continuous remodelling occurs, resulting in *relocation* or *drift*, illustrated by the hard palate, which subsides due to resorption of the nasal floor and concomitant deposition on the roof of the palate (Figures 3.9 and 3.11). Therefore, relocation and structural remodelling are closely related to each other. The downward movement of the hard palate in relation to fixed points overlying structures is therefore the result of two processes: relocation owing to remodelling growth and displacement of the maxilla. Knowledge of these separate processes is essential for a proper understanding of growth events and the effect

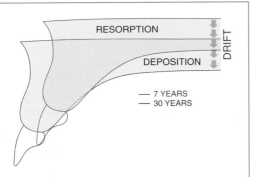

Figure 3.11 Illustration of relocation (drift) of the maxillary palate from 7 to 30 years of age. Resorption of the nasal floor and deposition on the roof of the palate.

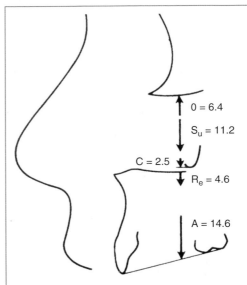

Figure 3.13 In 9 boys, the mean growth changes from the age of 4 years until adulthood (Björk and Skieller, 1977). Apposition at the floor of the orbit (O), sutural lowering of the maxilla (Su), apposition at the infrazygonatic crest (C), resorptive lowering of the nasal floor (Re), and increase in height of the alveolar process (A).

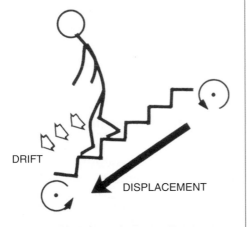

Figure 3.12 Schematic illustration of the combined effect of drift and displacement.

of various forms of orthodontic treatment. An orthopaedic force or fusion of sutures may prevent drift or even increase for the absence of displacement, illustrated in Figure 3.12. The downward movement by the staircase (displacement) can be stopped, but this does not exclude the possibility that the stick figure may continue or even increase its movement in that direction (drift).

Height The vertical growth of the middle face in relation to the anterior cranial base is the combined result of lowering of the maxilla by displacement and remodelling at the bone surfaces. Figure 3.13 summarises the average pattern observed by Björk and Skieller (1977). The displacement of the maxilla, classified as sutural lowering of the bone, creates space for an expansion of the nasal cavity and orbits. However, lowering of the orbital floor is limited by some bone deposition towards the orbits. The floor of the nasal cavity is continuously lowered owing to relocation. Vertical growth of the alveolar process is rapid during tooth eruption and exceeds the lowering of the roof of the palate three-fold.

Width Further expansion of the nasal cavity occurs by separation of the two maxillary bodies in the median suture (lateral displacement), and bone resorption on the lateral walls of the cavity. The separation of the two bodies is more marked posteriorly than anteriorly, suggesting that the lateral displacement includes a rotational movement of the bodies in relation to each other (Björk and Skieller, 1974). The transversal displacement exceeds the changes in the width of the dental arch. Consequently, adaptive changes in the width of the dental arch must compensate for the greater growth in width due to displacement.

Growth of the mandible

The two halves of the mandible, separated by a symphysis at birth, are fused into a single bone by the age of 1 to 2 years. The alveolar and muscle processes are poorly developed, so the shape of the mandible in the newborn is determined by its basal arch. Like the nasomaxillary complex, the mandible grows in size by periosteal remodelling in various degrees at different areas and at different ages, reflecting its growth pattern over the years. The tooth-bearing unit affects the growth in height. The role of the condylar cartilage in mandibular growth has been discussed over the years, and is still a subject of controversy. It has previously been claimed that it is an active growth centre, similar to the epiphyseal cartilages, thereby pushing the mandible forwards. The information at hand indicates that the condyle and its cartilage participate only in regional adaptive growth and are thus not a major growth centre for the whole mandible (Meikle, 1973).

Condylar cartilage

This secondary type of cartilage differs morphologically from epiphyseal and synchondrosal cartilage, which develop in membrane bones, but only at articulations that are mobile, or where the musculature sets up conditions of strain. The histo-morphological picture of the condylar cartilage varies from birth to adulthood, but the following layers can usually be seen (Thilander *et al.*, 1976):

■ a fibrous connective layer, richly vascularised at birth, but acquiring a dense fibrous character with increasing age (surface articular zone);
■ a highly cellular intermediate layer containing proliferating cells, which at a deeper level is a transitional stage between undifferentiated cells and cartilage cells (transitional or proliferating zone (PZ));
■ a zone with hypertrophic cartilage cells and a deeper layer of mineralised cartilage (hypertrophic zone);

■ a zone with bone ossification (bone formative zone).

The entire head of the condyle during the foetal stage and most of the condyle in the newborn consists of such cartilage. The cartilage decreases in thickness with age. At the age of 5 to 7 years, the whole cartilage layer is about half as thick as at the age of 6 months, and in young adult individuals only cartilage remnants are left. As the condyle is also a part of the ramus, the fibrous layer of condylar cartilage is in continuous connection with the periosteum of the ramus, and remodelling processes are seen in all components of the joint. The term 'condylar growth' is therefore misleading. According to Enlow (1990), 'ramus and condylar growth' is more correct. Only by recognizing that condylar cartilage is a product of the periosteum can the differences in cellular kinetics, structure and growth between condylar and epiphyseal cartilage be understood. This includes failure of the chondrocytes to divide and consequently the cells are not organized into parallel columns (Meikle, 2007).

Growth pattern of the mandible

Depth Like the maxillary complex, the mandible grows forwards and downwards because of two processes: by displacement of the whole bone and by relocation owing to remodelling at the ramus. The growth rate is especially marked at puberty, but a smaller peak at the ages round 7 years is also evident. The symphyseal part of the mandible, however, contributes little or nothing to its postnatal growth in length.

According to the 'active growth centre' theory, the mandible should be 'pushed' in an opposite direction to its upward growth path. According to the 'adaptive growth area' theory, however, the mandible as a whole should be 'pulled' in a forward direction due to its functional components, especially the jaw muscles group. These theories regarding displacement might be an academic point at issue, but are of interest in discussing the effect of an orthodontic appliance. Anyhow, the push or pull theory both creates conditions for periosteal remodelling at the ramus with deposition of bone on its

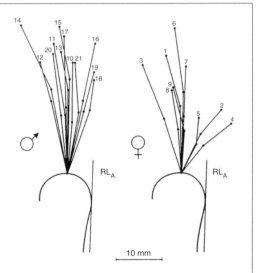

Figure 3.14 Variability in condylar growth from 3 years before to 3 years after puberty and measured by the implant method (Björk and Skieller, 1972). The values indicate case numbers of boys and girls. Note the curved paths of growth and variability in direction of growth relative to ramus line (RL$_A$).

posterior margin and simultaneous resorption along it anterior contours, i.e. relocation. This means that marked lengthening of the alveolar process will occur.

Height Growth in height enables the alveolar processes to adjust to the downward displacement of the mandibular body, depending on the direction and rate of the condylar growth, which shows great variability in individuals (Björk and Skieller, 1972) (Figure 3.14). In the majority of the children, the growth occurs in an anterior direction and varies by no less than 22 degrees, and the direction of growth also seems to vary from one period to another. Relative to the mandibular base, this growth is approximately 3 mm during childhood and around 5 mm during the pubertal growth spurt in contrast to the lower margin of the mandible, which contributes little to mandibular growth in height, but is the site of extensive remodelling related to rotational phenomenon associated with the growth of the jaws.

Björk's studies with metal markers in combination with X-ray cephalometry have above all served to illustrate the complexity of craniofacial growth, especially to the rotational changes exhibited by the jaws during growth. Rotation in this context means a change in the inclination of the mandibular body relative to the anterior cranial base (Figure 3.15). Anterior (upward) rotation will take place in subjects with a forward direction of condylar/rami growth, while in subject with a predominantly backward direction of that area, the mandible will rotate in a posterior (downward) direction. Coincident remodelling along its inferior margin reduces the apparent effect of this rotation on the facial morphology. Most individuals show an anterior (upward) rotation of the mandible, while a rotation of the maxilla is little or none.

Width Because of its early fusion, the mandibular symphysis plays little part in the width of the mandible. The two rami have a diverging shape in vertical section, which will contribute, not only in its growth in height, but also in its increase in width (Figure 3.16). A complex sequence of remodelling changes takes place during the growth of the mandibular body. Dental fixtures, placed in the mandibular jaws of growing pigs, clearly showed the increase in height of the alveolar processes, due to tooth eruption (Ödman *et al.,* 1991), and even changes in width of the jawbone (Thilander *et al.,* 1992). The fixture, originally placed in the buccal position, was in an inferior-lingual position 6 months later, due to bone remodelling and thereby giving an example of relocation in the displaced mandible.

Development of the dentoalveolar complex

The relation between the maxilla and the mandible is a result of developmental processes in which the main events are jaw growth and eruption of the teeth, resulting in contact between the jaws, i.e. occlusion. There is a close relation between the skeletal development of the jaws (maxilla and mandible) and the dentoalveolar complex. Interestingly, the dentoalveolar structures do not seem essential for the development of the basal parts of the facial frame, but they appear to possess the potential

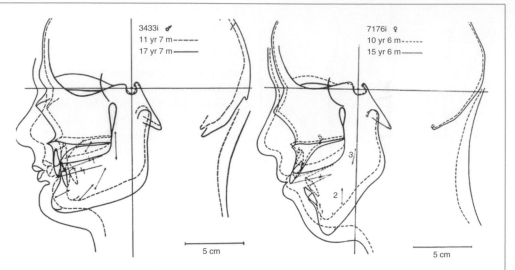

Figure 3.15 Tracings of cephalograms superimposed on the skull base. To the left, anterior (upward) rotation from 11 years and 7 months to 17 years and 7 months of age. To the right, posterior (downward rotation) from 10 years and 6 months to 15 years and 6 months of age.

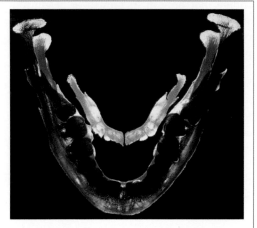

Figure 3.16 Development of the mandible with its complex sequence of remodelling changes.

for counteracting slight discrepancies in the development of the jaw relations, thus maintaining acceptable relations between the maxillary and mandibular dental arches (Solow, 1980).

The formation of the maxillary and mandibular alveolar processes depends on inductive influences from the developing teeth. In absence of teeth, the alveolar bone fails to develop. The mechanisms and factors that control the development of the dentition differ from those of the facial bones. Tooth development is under a very strict genetic control, including the

characteristic form of the teeth as well as cell differentiation and matrix deposition by the odontoblasts, ameloblasts and cementoblasts. The progress in molecular biology and gene technology has resulted in a better understanding of those processes (Thesleff, 1995). Genetic and environmental processes show a great deal of individual variation, and consequently remarkable co-ordination of different events is necessary for development of a 'normal' Angle Class I occlusion. Failure in one part may lead to different types of malocclusions, described in Chapter 2.

Eruption of the teeth

The development of the dentition is a long process. It starts during the embryonic period when the first primary teeth are initiated, and continues to the complete development of the third permanent molars during young adulthood. The tooth starts to move inside the bone when root development has started, and during continuous eruption it reaches occlusion. However, it should be stressed that eruption still continues after completed root development, and consequently, slow eruption can be seen even in adults (Iseri and Solow, 1996; Thilander *et al.*, 2001).

The *mechanisms* involved in tooth eruption are not fully understood. It is not known

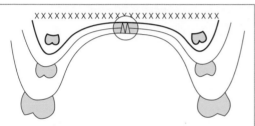

Figure 3.17 The palatal height increases during tooth eruption.

what initiates eruption and what causes the movement of the tooth to the oral cavity and subsequently into occlusion. Furthermore, the process in shedding the primary tooth for its permanent successor is very complex, because it involves metabolic and structural changes in the tooth as well as in all tissues surrounding the tooth germ. However, it has been suggested that the biological regulatory mechanisms for tooth eruption may be linked to the dental follicle. In addition, the role of the periodontal ligament (PDL) has also been discussed in the continuing eruption after emergence into the oral cavity.

During tooth eruption, the increase in alveolar processes is rapid, illustrated by palatal height (Figure 3.17). A longitudinal study of dentoalveolar development (Thilander, 2009) clearly showed a slow continuous increase in palatal height, even from 16 to 31 years of age. This increase is full of the following inconsistences: with premolars and molars in occlusion, no further increase should occur;

continuous remodelling of the palate with bone deposition orally should decrease this distance; as should tooth wear with increasing age. Thus, the increase of palatal height (0.1 mm/year) might be an effect of a slow continuous eruption and seems to indicate an important role in the eruption mechanism. This knowledge is of importance in explaining the infraposition of an implant-supported crown as a continuous eruption of its adjacent teeth (Figure 3.18) (Thilander *et al.*, 2001).

Chronology of primary and permanent teeth

Certain differences in *primary* tooth eruption exist between racial groups. European and American babies seem to be the earliest, but no differences have been found after the age of 1 to 2 years. In a Swedish population, the mean eruption time of the first tooth (mandibular medial incisor) is 8.1 months and the last one (maxillary second molar) at 29.1 months, without distinction between sexes (Lysell *et al.*, 1969). However, individual differences in time and order exist.

Eruption of the permanent teeth has been recorded in large samples of schoolchildren from different ethnic groups with help of panoramic radiographs. Standards of dental development based on various stages of tooth formation are at present available for many population groups. Studies in Scandinavian populations show high agreement and Table 3.1 presents the mean age of the emergence of the different teeth

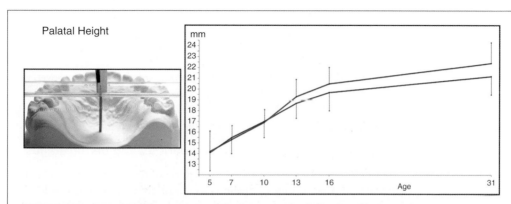

Figure 3.18 Diagram showing mean increase in palatal height (mm) from 5 to 31 years of age; males (blue line) and females (red line).

Table 3.1 Time and order of emergence of permanent teeth (based on data of Helm and Seidler, 1974).

Girls							
Maxilla				**Mandible**			
	−2SD	Mean	+2SD		−2SD	Mean	+2SD
Tooth				Tooth			
I1	5.6	**7.0**	8.4	I1	4.7	**6.0**	7.3
I2	6.0	**7.8**	9.6	I2	5.5	**7.1**	8.7
C	8.3	**10.8**	13.3	C	7.5	**9.6**	11.7
P1	7.5	**10.1**	12.7	P1	7.4	**10.0**	12.6
P2	8.2	**11.0**	13.8	P2	8.1	**11.0**	13.9
M1	4.8	**6.1**	7.4	M1	4.8	**6.0**	7.2
M2	9.5	**11.9**	14.3	M2	9.0	**11.4**	13.8

Boys							
Maxilla				**Mandible**			
	−2SD	Mean	+2SD		−2SD	Mean	+2SD
Tooth				Tooth			
I1	5.7	**7.2**	8.7	I1	4.9	**6.2**	7.5
I2	6.5	**8.2**	9.9	I2	5.6	**7.4**	9.2
C	9.1	**11.5**	13.9	C	8.3	**10.6**	12.8
P1	7.7	**10.6**	13.5	P1	7.7	**10.7**	13.6
P2	8.5	**11.4**	14.3	P2	8.6	**11.5**	14.4
M1	4.9	**6.3**	7.7	M1	4.8	**6.2**	7.6
M2	9.9	**12.4**	14.9	M2	9.3	**11.9**	14.5

Order of emergence of permanent teeth				
maxilla	M1 I1	I2	P1 P2	C M2
mandible	M1/I1 I2		C/P1 P2	P2 M2
year	6 7	8 9	10 11	12 13

Key: Mean age, very early (−2SD) and very late (+2SD) ages. I1 = central incisor; I2 = lateral incisor; C = canine; P1 = 1st premolar; P2 = 2nd premolar; M1 = 1st molar; M2 = 2nd molar.

in Danish children (Helm and Seidler, 1974). There are developmental differences between boys and girls, as well as between individual children. Some are 'early' and some are 'late' throughout. Within two standard deviations (SD) of the mean, emergence age is usually considered as 'normal'. For example, the mean age of the maxillary canine in girls is 10.8 years, but the normal range (2SD) is as large as 5 years. This large individual variation must be kept in mind for orthodontic diagnosis and treatment planning of children. Moreover, there exist differences between the jaws; for example, the mandibular canine erupts earlier than the canine in the maxilla (Table 3.1).

Dentition periods and dental stages

Due to eruption of the primary and permanent teeth, the dentition periods are divided into the primary, the mixed and the permanent dentition. The time of the mixed dentition can be divided in three different periods as well:

Table 3.2 Classification of age groups into developmental periods, based on dental stages (DS).

Age groups		Developmental periods	DS
Year	Range		
5	4.2–5.8	Primary dentition	DS 02
7	6.6–8.2	Early mixed dentition	DS1M0, DS1M1, DS2M0
10	9.5–11.2	Late mixed dentition	DS2M1, DS3M1
13	12.3–13.8	Early permanent dentition	DS3M2, DS4M1
16	14.9–17.1	Permanent dentition	DS4M2

Key: DS 01 = primary dentition erupting;
 DS 02 = primary dentition complete;
 DS 1 = early mixed dentition with incisors erupting;
 DS 2 = mixed dentition with incisors fully erupted;
 DS 3 = late mixed dentition with canines and premolars erupting;
 DS 4 = permanent dentition with canines and premolars fully erupted;
 M1 = first molars fully erupted;
 M2 = second molars fully erupted (Thilander, 2009).

1 the first transitional period during which the first molars emerge and erupt, the primary incisors are shed, and the permanent incisors emerge and erupt (early mixed dentition);

2 the intertransitional period, which on average lasts approximately 2 years;

3 the second transitional period during which the primary canines and molars are shed, and the permanent canines, premolars and second molars emerge (late mixed dentition). This is a period of rapid change in a child's dentition, which lasts on average for 2 years. During this relatively short time, 12 primary teeth are shed and 16 new teeth emerge into the oral cavity. This is a period when many malocclusions are manifested.

The concept of dental stages, according to tooth emergence status, was introduced by Björk *et al.* (1964), and defined as follows:

• primary teeth erupting (DS 01) or fully erupted (DS 02);
• canines and premolars erupting (DS 3) or fully erupted (DS 4);
• first molars erupting (DS M0) and fully erupted (DS M1);
• second molars (DS M2) and third molars (DS M3) fully erupted.

Dental stages are very useful in clinical work, both in diagnosis and in treatment planning.

Classification of age groups and dental stages in Swedish children between 5 and 16 year of age are shown in Table 3.2 (Thilander, 2009). The great differences between chronologic age and dental stages are obvious.

Development of the dental arches and occlusion

The development of the human dentition is a continuous process, as asserted already by Friel (1927), and his statement has later been verified by longitudinal studies (Baume, 1950; Moorrees, 1959; Sillman, 1965; Bishara *et al.,* 1995). Furthermore, a collection of dry skulls (van der Linden and Duterloo, 1976), and an atlas of radiographic X-rays of the developing dentition (Duterloo, 1991) can clearly demonstrate that dentoalveolar development is an extremely complex biological process. Finally, a longitudinal study of Swedes with normal/ideal dentitions, without any history of orthodontic treatment, illustrates the great morphological variations within the dental arches between the ages of 5 and 31 years (Thilander, 2009).

■ The arch length in the posterior segment decreases between 7 and 13 years (maxilla: 1 mm; mandible: 3 mm), due to differences between the mesiodistal crown diameters of the primary and permanent teeth, known as leeway space (Figure 3.19). After that period, a

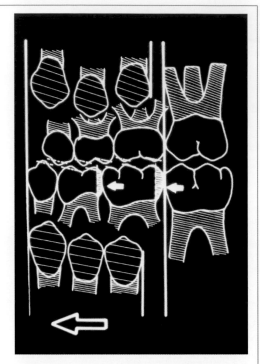

Figure 3.19 The mesiodistal tooth widths of deciduous molars are larger than the permanent teeth (premolars). Usually the sum of the primary tooth widths is greater than that of their permanent successors. Therefore, when these primary teeth fall out, there is usually a slight amount of space of about 2 to 3 mm per side in the mandible and 1 to 2 mm in the maxilla.

followed by a continuous decrease to adult ages. The intermolar width in the two jaws followed the above pattern.

The development of the dental arches, expressed as the circumference, is dependent on a decrease in the posterior segments (leeway space and mesial migration), an increase in the anterior segment (due to erupting incisors in proclined position), and an increase of the arch width. Despite these developmental changes, no change in the arch perimeter, mesial of the first molars, occurs between 5 and 31 years of age in the maxilla, contrary to a decrease of 4 mm in the mandible. Even in 'ideal' dental arches, the physiological migration may have an influence on tooth position in the ideal Angle Class I occlusion. All those developmental changes should be considered in orthodontic treatment planning and in evaluation of the post-retention development.

Growth of soft tissues

Muscular growth

In most mammal muscles, the number of muscle fibres does not increase after embryonic differentiation of the tissue, indicating genetic control. Therefore, subsequent growth of a muscle mainly will occur in terms of fibre size due to an increase in myofibrils within the fibre (Goldspink, 1974), which means that post-embryonic growth of a muscle results from hyperplasia rather than hypertrophy. The fibres grow at their ends, where new sarcomeres add to the existing myofibrils, induced by mechanical factors such as passive stretching, rather than by neural reflexes.

Apart from a remodelling response in the bone tissue, further adaptation between muscle tissue and the skeletal framework can take place through changes in the origin of the muscles and their insertion at the bone surface, or through the replacement of muscle fibres by tendons. It is well known from sports physiology, that certain forms of exercises are more effective than others in inducing this hypertrophy and

further decrease occurs. The anterior segment increases between 5 and 10 years (maxilla: 6 mm; mandible: 4 mm) owing to eruption of the incisors into a proclined position, then followed by a continuous decrease up to 31 years of age. Eruption of the incisors even involved an increase of the arch depth. A continuous slow decrease (1–2 mm in both jaws) after the age of 13 years indicates a slow mesial physiological migration of the occlusion.

■ The arch width shows different pattern in the jaws. The intercanine width in the maxilla increases up to 16 years (4 mm). In the mandible, an increase of the same degree was recorded up to the age of 10 years, and then

thus increasing the contractile force of the muscles, which may in turn influence the skeletal morphology. Considering the craniofacial area, it has been shown that bilateral hypertrophy of the masseter muscle is linked with changes in the jaw angle. Furthermore, animals fed on a hard diet show local thickening of the bone in the region of the muscle insertion of the mandible compared with a group fed an identical but softened diet (Kiliaridis, 1986). Changes in craniofacial morphology have even been recorded in patients with hypotonic musculature (Kiliaridis *et al.*, 1989).

Function or movements of the mandible certainly have an influence on facial morphology. A functional phenomenon, related to the physiological rest position of the mandible, may change the relation between the jaws, especially in a functional crossbite. When the mandible is guided laterally from a retroposition (RP) into an intercuspal position (ICP), a 'forced posterior crossbite' will develop; and when guided anteriorly, a 'forced anterior crossbite' will develop. Taken together, observations suggest an independence of muscle tissue and surrounding structures, so that muscle growth is relatively well synchronized with the growth of the skeletal framework. Although bone tissues remodel as a response to functional load, it has been reported that the skeletal muscle is one of the most adaptable tissue in the body.

Soft tissue profile

Changes in the soft tissue profile with age follow the growth in the underlying hard tissue, but they are not directly correlated to each other. Increase in facial height and sagittal mandibular growth may diminish the convexity of the profile with age, especially in males. Our subjective impression of changes in the soft tissue profile is strongly influenced by growth of the nose. Nasal growth mainly occurs in the anterior-inferior direction, particularly during the pubertal growth spurt, with marked changes in size as well as in shape (Posen, 1967). The lip profile also changes during childhood and adolescence, partly due to changes in skeletal growth and partly owing to changes of the dentition, especially the incisor inclination. Since most changes of the soft tissues occur during the puberty growth spurt, it is difficult to predict the soft tissue profile at an early age.

Prediction of growth

Different methods have been presented, but due to the complexity of the craniofacial growth pattern, the reliability of the predictions has been low and the confidence intervals too wide to be of clinical interest in orthodontics (Houston *et al.*, 1979). Certain parameters have been shown to follow a stable pattern and can therefore be predicted with reasonable certainty (e.g. body height). On the other hand, it is both difficult and impracticable to estimate the future growth pattern of a skeletal malocclusion in a growing child, which should involve a large number of children with an untreated malocclusion, matched with controls, and followed during a long observation period. Such a project is of great academic interest but is, due to ethical reasons, hardly realizable. Growth is not a random process. From a clinical point of view, it is important to remember that the roughly 10% of children who have a strongly deviating growth pattern, are also those whose growth is most difficult to predict (Walker, 1972).

Conclusions

The aim of this chapter is to describe the complexity of craniofacial growth and development. Both skeletal and dentofacial components must co-operate to result in a 'normal face' with 'ideal occlusion', a lifelong process starting already during the prenatal period. However, in roughly 70% of a population, something goes wrong in this cycle, resulting in divergences in the relation between the jaws, within the jaws, or related to a single tooth. Therefore, the cause for the defect in question should be analysed at the examination to make a differential diagnosis, which is of great importance in the treatment planning.

REFERENCES

Baume, L. (1950) Physiological tooth migration and its significance for the development of the occlusion. J Dent Res 29: 331–337.

Bishara, S.E., Khadivi, P. and Jacobsen, J.R. (1995) Changes in tooth-arch length relationships from deciduous to permanent dentition: a longitudinal study. Am J Orthod and Dentofac Orthop 108: 607–613.

Bjoerk, A., Krebs, A. and Solow, B. (1964) A method of epidemiological registration of malocclusion. Acta Odont Scand 22: 27–41.

Björk, A. and Skieller, V. (1972) Facial development and tooth eruption. Am J Orthod 62: 339–383.

Björk, A. and Skieller, V. (1974) Growth in width of the maxilla studied by the implant method. Scand J Plast Reconstr Surg 8: 26–33.

Björk, A. and Skieller, V. (1977) Growth of the maxilla in three dimensions as revealed radiographically by the implant method. Brit J Orthod 4: 53–64.

Bondevik, O. (2012) Dentofacial changes in adults. A longitudinal cephalometric study in 22–33 and 33–43 year olds. J Orofac Orthop 73: 277–288.

Brundtland, G.H., Liestöl, K. and Wallöe, L. (1980) Height, weight and menarcheal age of Oslo schoolchildren at the last 60 years. Ann Human Biol 7: 307–322.

Capulli, M., Paone, R. and Rucci, N. (2014) Osteoblast and osteocyte. Arch Biochem Biophys 561: 3–12.

Civitelli, R. (2008) Cell–cell communication in the osteoblast/osteocyte lineage. Arch Biochem Biophys 473: 188–192.

Demirjian, A. and Godstein, H. (1976) New systems for dental maturity based on seven and four teeth. Ann Human Biol 3: 411–421.

Duterloo, H.S. (1991) *An Atlas of Dentition in Childhood Orthodontic Diagnosis and panoramic Radiology*. London, Wolfe Publishing Ltd.

Enlow, D. H. (1990) *Facial Growth*, 3rd edition. W.B. Saunders Co, Philadelphia.

Ferguson, M.W. (1991) The orofacial region. In: *Textbook of Fetal and perinatal Pathology* (Eds J.S. Wigglesworth and D.B. Singer). Blackwell, Oxford.

Friel, S. (1927) Occlusion. Observations on its development from infancy to old age. *Trans First Int Orthod Congress*. C.V. Mosby, St Louis, pp. 138–159.

Goldspink, G. (1974) Development of muscles. In: *Differentiation and Growth of Cells in Vertebrate Tissues* (Ed. G. Goldspink). Chapman & Hall, London.

Helm, S. and Seidler, B. (1974) Timing of permanent tooth emergency in Danish children. Community Dent Oral Epidemiol 2: 122–129.

Houston, J.W.B., Miller, J.C. and Tanner, J.M. (1979) Prediction of the timing of the adolescent growth spurt from ossification events in handwrist films. Brit J Orthod 6: 145–152.

Huggare, J. (1995) Craniocervical junction as a focus for craniofacial growth studies. Acta Odont Scand 53: 186–191.

Iseri, H. and Solow, B. (1996) Continued eruption of maxillary incisors and first molars in girls from 9 to 25 years, studied by the implant method. Eur J Orthod 18: 245–256.

Kiliaridis, S. (1986) Masticatory muscle function and craniofacial morphology. Swed Dent J, Suppl 36: 1–55.

Kiliaridis, S., Mejersjö. C. and Thilander, B. (1989) Muscle function and craniofacial morphology: a clinical study in patients with myotonic dystrophy. Eur J Orthod 11: 131–138.

Lecanda, F., Warlow, P.M. *et al.* (2000) Connexin43 deficiency causes delayed ossification, craniofacial abnormalities, and osteoblast dysfunction. J Cell Biol 151: 931–944.

Lysell, L., Magnusson, B. and Thilander, B. (1969) Relations between the times of eruption of primary and permanent teeth.

A longitudinal study. Acta Odont Scand 27: 271–281.

Meikle, M.C. (1973) The role of the condyle in the postnatal growth of the mandible. Am J Orthod 64: 50–62.

Meikle, M.C. (2007) Remodeling of the dentofacial skeleton. J Dent Res 86: 12–24.

Moorrees, C. (1959) *The Dentition of the Growing Child: a longitudinal study of dental development between 3 and 18 years of age.* Harvard University Press, Cambridge, MA.

Melsen, B. (1974) The cranial base. Acta Odont Scand 32: Suppl 62.

Moss, L.M. (1962) The functional matrix. In: *Vistas of Orthdontics* (Eds B.L. Kraus and R.A. Riedel). Lee and Febiger, Philadelphia.

Ödman, J., Gröndahl, K., Lekholm, U. and Thilander, B. (1991) The effect of osseointegrated implants on the dento-alveolar development. A clinical and radiographic study in growing pigs. Eur J Orthod 13: 279–286.

Persson, M. (1973) Structure and growth of facial sutures. Odont Rev 24, Suppl 26.

Persson, M. and Thilander, B. (1977) Palatal suture closure in man from 15 to 35 years of age. Am J Orthod 72: 42–52.

Persson, M., Magnusson, B. and Thilander, B. (1978) Sutural closure in rabbit and man: a morphological and histochemical study. J Anat 125: 313–321.

Posen, J.M. (1967) A longitudinal study of the growth of the nose. Am J Orthod 53: 746–756.

Ransjö, M., Sahli, J. and Lie, A. (2003) Expression of connexin43 mRNA in microisolated murine osteoclasts and regulation of bone resorption *in vitro* by gap junction inhibitors. Biochem Biophys Res Commun 303: 1179–1185.

Roberts, S.J., van Gastel, N., Carmeliet, G., Leuyten, F.P. (2015) Uncovering the periosteum for skeletal regeneration: the stem cell that lies beneath. Bone 70: 10–18.

Sarnat, B.G. Wexler, M.R. (1968) Postnatal growth of the nose and face after resection of septal cartilage in the rabbit. Oral Surg Oral med Oral Pathol 26: 712–727.

Scott, J.H. (1962) The growth of the craniofacial skeleton. Irish J Med Science 428: 276–286.

Sillman, J.H. (1965) Some aspects of individual dental development: longitudinal study from birth to 25 years. Am J Orthod 51: 1–25.

Solow B. (1980) The dentoalveolar compensatory mechanism: background and clinical implications. Br J Orthod 7: 145–161.

Solow, B. and Tallgren, A. (1976) Head posture and craniofacial morphology. Am J of Physical Anthropology 44: 417–435.

Stenström, S. and Thilander, B. (1970) Effects of nasal septal cartilage resections on young guinea pigs. Plast Reconstr Surg 45: 160–170.

Ten Cate A.R. (Ed.) (1980) Embryology of the head, face, and oral cavity. In: *Oral Histology.* Mosby Co, St Louis.

Thesleff, I. (1995) The teeth. In: *Embryos, Genes and Birth Defects* (Ed. P. Thorogood). Wiley & Sons, UK.

Thilander, B. and Ingervall, B. (1973) The human sphenooccipital synchondrosis. II: A histological and microradiographic study of its growth. Acta Odont Scand 31: 323–334.

Thilander, B., Carlsson, G. and Ingervall, B. (1976) Postnatal development of the human temporomandibular joint. I: A histological study. Acta Odont Scand 34: 117–126.

Thilander, B., Ödman, J., Gröndahl, K. and Lekholm, U. (1992) Aspects on osseointegrated implants inserted in growing jaws. A biometric and radiographic study in the young pig. Eur J Orthod 14: 99–109.

Thilander, B., Ödman, J. and Lekholm, U. (2001) Orthodontic aspects on the use of oral implants in adolescents: a 10-year follow-up study. Eur J Orthod 23: 715–731.

Thilander, B., Persson, M. and Adolfsson, U. (2005) Roentgen-cephalometric standards for a Swedish population. A longitudinal study between the ages of 5 and 31 years of age. Eur J Orthod 27: 370–389.

Thilander, B. (2009) Dento-alveolar development in subjects with normal occlusion. A longitudinal study between the ages of 5 and 31 years. Eur J Orthod 31: 109–120.

Walker, G. (1972) A new approach to the analysis of craniofacial morphology and growth. Am J Orthod 61: 221–230.

van der Linden, F.P.G.M. and Duterloo, H.S. (1976) *Development of the Human Dentition – an atlas*. Harper & Row Publishers, Hagerstown Maryland.

Zappittelli, T. and Aubin, J.E. (2014) The 'Connexin' between bone cells and skeletal functions. J Cell Biochem 115: 1646–1658.

CHAPTER 4
Diagnostic examinations

Krister Bjerklin and Lars Bondemark

Key topics

- General examination of the orthodontic patient
- Interview for the anamnesis
- Extra oral examination
- Intra oral examination
- Functional examination
- Examinations at different dental developmental stages/ages and of adults

Learning objectives

- To perform a comprehensive orthodontic examination for a basis to make an orthodontic diagnosis, which in turn forms a cornerstone for the treatment plan
- To know how to assess examinations at different dental stages/ages, including adults

Essential Orthodontics, First Edition. Birgit Thilander, Krister Bjerklin and Lars Bondemark.
© 2018 John Wiley & Sons Ltd. Published 2018 by John Wiley & Sons Ltd.

Introduction

Usually, the first meeting between the clinician and a patient starts with an interview with the patient, discussing general and oral health status (past and present), any medication, the chief complaint, followed by the patient's attitude towards an eventual orthodontic treatment. When it comes to child patients, it is important that one or, preferably, both parents are present during the interview and examination. After the interview is performed, the clinical examination is assessed. The clinical examination includes an extra- and intra oral analysis of morphology and function. Often, the clinical examination has to be supplemented with further analyses using extra- and intra oral photographs, study casts (model analysis) and radiographs. The results from the interview, clinical examination and the supplementary analyses will constitute a solid basis for a comprehensive orthodontic diagnosis, which in turn forms a cornerstone for the treatment plan.

Examination of cleft-lip-palate children and children with syndromes and disabilities are not included in this chapter. These children have an individualised examination programme depending on the individual condition and are carefully examined during the first week after birth by specialist teams in which, for example, plastic surgeons, oral surgeons, speech therapists, child psychologists and orthodontists are included.

Interview and anamnesis

To provide the best conditions for an interview, it is important that the conversation takes place in an undisturbed environment, there is ample time and that the dentist actively listens to the patient and lets the patient express what has brought her/him to the clinic. It may also be helpful for the dentist to use a checklist in order to avoid losing important information (Figure 4.1).

In the interview with the patient, it is essential to consider the general health conditions, possible medication and whether the patient suffers from allergies. It is also relevant to include questions of family history since malocclusions, growth and development may be expressions of genetic patterns.

Questions on the general health, with special emphasis on diseases and medication are valuable, since diseases causing altered metabolism may affect growth and tissue reactions. Furthermore, medication with anti-inflammatory drugs can interact with bone turnover, which is important in orthodontic treatment. Allergies may affect the mode of breathing and respiratory capacity. It can also be noted that an orthodontic appliance may contain various metals and composites, which although rare, can cause contact allergies. For example, if the dentist is aware that the patient is allergic to nickel before the treatment begins, nickel-containing materials like stainless steel, which is a frequently used component in orthodontic appliance, can be replaced with other materials, to avoid the risk of allergic reactions.

It is also important to ask the patient about dental trauma and experience of headache. Frequency of headache can be rated on a 5-point scale: never, a few times per year, every month, every week and every day (List *et al.*, 1999).

Considering child patients, the psychological development and previous experience of dental treatment has to be stressed, especially when deciding the start and mode of treatment. Many children have received very little dental care, and it can be a delicate task for the dentist to determine how well these patients can tolerate orthodontic treatment for 1.5 to 2.5 years. Furthermore, often there are situations where a child patient is very eager to start the treatment, but the assessment is that the child's present psychological and social development makes it better to perform the treatment later.

Extra oral examination

The examination starts with the patient standing in order to study the body physiognomy (size and nutrition state). The body height can be measured in cases where the growth is regarded important for the treatment outcome.

The face is then observed in both frontal and lateral view to assess symmetry and harmony (van der Linden and Boersma, 1987). The best way to examine the face is to sit opposite the

Anamnesis
general health
allergy
headache, way of breathing, snoring
sucking habits, nail biting
earlier trauma to the face or teeth
earlier orthodontic treatment
earlier extraction of primary or permanent teeth
heredity, orthodontic treatment or malocclusions in the family
Extra oral examination
face symmetry, face profile, face harmonious
way of swallowing, way of breathing
soft tissue
lip closure
palpation of jaw muscles
maximal jaw opening, pain or irregular movement
temporomandibular jaws, pain, clicking or other sound
Intra oral examination
soft tissues including tongue and frenulae
tonsils and adenoides
oral hygiene, caries activity
primary and permanent teeth: number and conditions
palpation of maxillary canines
occlusion: sagitally, vertically and transversally
overjet, overbite
space circumstances in the dental arches
tooth discrepancy: agenesis, tipping, rotation, infraocclusion, impaction
midlines in the maxilla and the mandible
function forced bite anteriorly or transversally
palpation of jaw muscles: masseter and temporalis muscles bilaterally

Figure 4.1 Check-list for registrations at the examination.

patient with the patient's and dentist's heads at the same level and the patient holding the head in a normal relaxed head position.

Examination of the frontal view can disclose asymmetry of eyes, nose and chin. The dental midlines of the maxilla and mandible are determined in relation to the facial midline. For determination of midline discrepancies between the jaws and the facial midline, it is recommended to have the patient lying down flat in the dental chair and the examiner sitting behind the patient's head asking the patient to smile. The midline deviation has to be greater than 1 mm to be registered.

The lateral view of the face exposes the face profile and the profile can be characterised into straight, convex and concave profiles (Figure 4.2). Most patients have a straight to slightly convex profile. The prominence of the nose and chin in relation to the profile can also be noted, as well as the texture of the lips. When the patient is in a relaxed position, it is also important to observe whether the lips cover the incisors, i.e. competent lip closure or whether an incomplete lip closure is apparent (Figure 4.3). In an incomplete lip closure situation, there is an increased risk of trauma to the maxillary incisors (Dimberg *et al.*, 2015; Petti, 2015).

In more specific cases, it can also be noteworthy to check the nasio-labial angle, since this angle often reflects the incisor positions, i.e. a large nasio-labial angle may imply

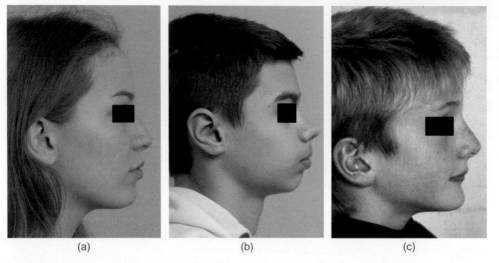

Figure 4.2 A straight profile (a), a convex (b), and a concave profile (c).

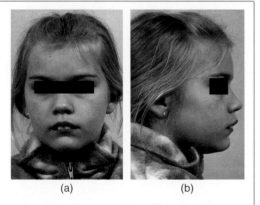

Figure 4.3 A 9-year-old girl with incomplete lip closure because of a large overjet (a,b).

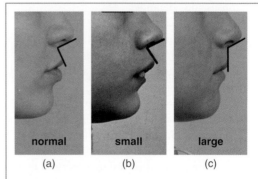

Figure 4.4 Normal (a), small (b), and large nasio-labial angle (c).

retroclined maxillary incisors and small angle proclined incisors (Figure 4.4). In addition, if the mentolabial fold is marked (Figure 4.5), this should be noted because a marked mentolabial fold indicates high muscular strain on mandibular incisors.

The vertical dimension of the face may also be examined. Often the vertical height of the face is divided into three parts: the top part from the hairline to where the nose begins, the middle part is the vertical height of the nose, and the lowest part corresponds to the height of the upper and lower lips plus the chin height (Figure 4.6). Analysing the vertical dimension

can give the dentist information about whether the patient represents a short or a long vertical face (Figure 4.7).

Extra oral coloured photographs are recommended and are helpful in assessing the examination of the lateral and frontal view of the face. The usual views are at rest and smiling: full facial frontal, facial three-quarters view, and facial profile (Figure 4.8).

Functional examination

The functional extra oral examination consists of identifying breathing and swallowing patterns as well as examination of mandibular

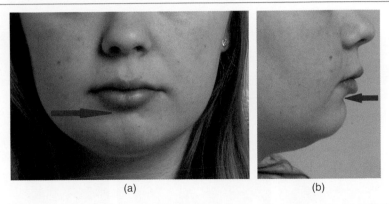

(a)   (b)

Figure 4.5 A marked mentolabial fold (arrow) indicating high muscular strain on the mandibular incisors. Frontal view (a) and lateral view (b).

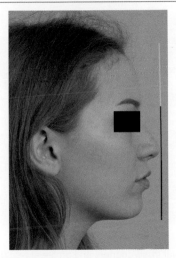

Figure 4.6 A normal vertically proportioned face, that is, one-third from the hairline to the nose (yellow line), one-third is the length of the nose (red line), and one-third is the lips and chin (black line).

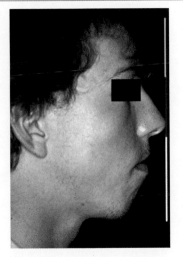

Figure 4.7 A long vertical face: note the increased vertical height of the lower third of the face (white line).

jaw movement, temporomandibular joint and muscle function.

Breathing and swallowing patterns are of interest, since abnormal patterns often imply altered muscle function that may contribute to tooth movements and can influence growth and development. Mouth breathing can occur for many different reasons, such as narrow nasal passages due to enlarged tonsils or adenoids. Mouth breathing in the long term may result in alterations of growth and development, while an abnormal swallowing pattern (e.g. swallowing with tongue pressure on teeth) may result in spacing of teeth or an open bite in children.

Abnormal speech should be noted, even if the evidence is insufficient for the interdependence between speech and malocclusions. However, occasionally when a patient has a very large tongue or when general spacing exists with large diastema between the teeth, speech is claimed to be affected.

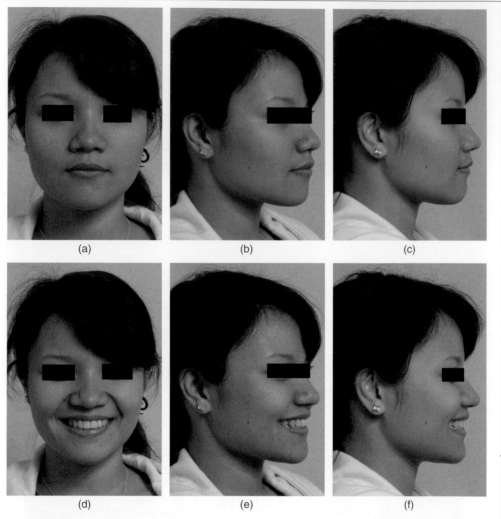

Figure 4.8 Extra oral photos with the usual views, i.e. frontal, facial three-quarters and profile at rest (a–c) and smiling (d–f).

To investigate eventual temporomandibular disorder (TMD) pain in adolescents, asking two questions can be recommended to detect those who have TMD pain:

1 Do you have pain in your temples, face, temporomandibular joint or jaws once a week or more?
2 Do you have pain when you open your mouth wide or chew, once a week or more?

If the answer is 'yes' to one of the questions, it is recommended to further examine the patient (Nilsson *et al.*, 2006). Such examination is recommended to follow the diagnostic criteria for temporomandibular disorders (DC/TMD) (Schiffman *et al.*, 2014). Nevertheless, at least registrations of mandibular movement capacity and palpation of the temporomandibular joints (TMJ) and masticatory muscles should be performed. Any noise from the TMJs during jaw movement is also recorded as well as palpation of the TMJs laterally and posteriorly, and the presence of pain is noted (Magnusson and Helkimo, 2009).

Normally the maximum jaw opening without pain should be at least 36 mm at the age of 6 to 7 years and a minimum of 41 mm after the age of 12 years.

An evaluation of the occlusion should also be included in the functional examination, and this primarily concerns whether lateral or forward directed forced guidance of the mandible is evident by an early intermaxillary abnormal contact when the bite is closing.

Intra oral examination

The intra oral examination starts with inspecting the oral mucosa, tonsils, possible adenoids and frenula, stage of dental development (number of primary and permanent teeth), signs of earlier trauma, oral hygiene, caries activity and amount of dental restorations, as well as gingival and periodontal conditions. Particularly in adults, the periodontal status including the gingival pockets should be carefully registered. Previous or newly taken intra oral radiographs or panoramic radiographs can be useful for determining the periodontal status.

The dental status or classifications of malocclusions in sagittal, vertical and transversal relation shall always be registered (see Chapter 2). To classify the occlusion in the three planes – determine the arch form, analyse the positions of individual teeth and measure the interproximal contact point discrepancies and space conditions in the jaw – it may often be easier to use a model analysis. Therefore, the clinical examination is usually supplemented by assessing impressions for study models. Moreover, coloured intra oral photographs can be excellent instruments to survey the intra oral status of a patient. Normally, five intra oral photographs are taken: frontal occlusion, right and left buccal occlusion, occlusal views of maxillary and mandibular arch (Figure 4.9).

Model analysis

Models for analyses can be made by impression for plaster models or by three-dimensional (3D) intra oral scanning. The requirements for good models are that they should cover all teeth, the palate and alveolar processes (Figure 4.10). Normally, the relation between the jaws should be in centric occlusion. Model analyses are also valuable for longitudinal evaluations of development and check-ups of treatment results.

Radiographic analysis

The use of radiographic investigations (e.g. intra oral, panoramic and lateral head radiograph, as well as 3D imaging) are unequalled for many situations, but should be based on strict individual needs and depend on what is found in the clinical examination. Radiographs should only be used when a clear individual indication exists, and the benefit gained for the patient with the radiograph must be weighed against the dosage of the X-ray (risk). Moreover, radiographs should not be used to obtain information for use in the future, for instance, for follow-ups, expected spontaneous corrections or to wait for the best time to start a treatment.

Intra oral radiographs can be used in any part of the mouth. For example, in the anterior region for evaluating the root form of incisors, estimating root length before and after treatment, i.e. in-detail study of possible root resorptions during or after treatment. Moreover, intra oral radiographs are valuable in locating unerupted teeth or ectopically positioned maxillary canines and local pathology. To determine the location of teeth or the inter-relationship between unerupted teeth and adjacent roots often requires at least two radiographs taken at different angles (parallax technique). Furthermore, eruption obstacles and supernumerary teeth, such as mesiodens, can be disclosed by intra oral radiographs.

Panoramic radiographs reveal an overall view of the presence, position and morphology of unerupted teeth and serve in the analysis of tooth development patterns, restorative status and the presence of pathology in the jaws, including maxillary sinus and the mandibular ramus and condyle (Bondemark *et al.*, 2006). However, it can be stressed that the panoramic radiograph should not be assessed for screening of asymptomatic patients.

Lateral head radiographs are often helpful as a supplement to the clinical diagnosis. From a lateral head radiograph, a cephalometric analysis can be carried out to determine the sagittal and vertical positions of the jaws in relation to the cranial base, as well as to classify the discrepancies that may exist between the jaws and to make differential diagnosis with respect to skeletal and dentoalveolar discrepancies. Thus,

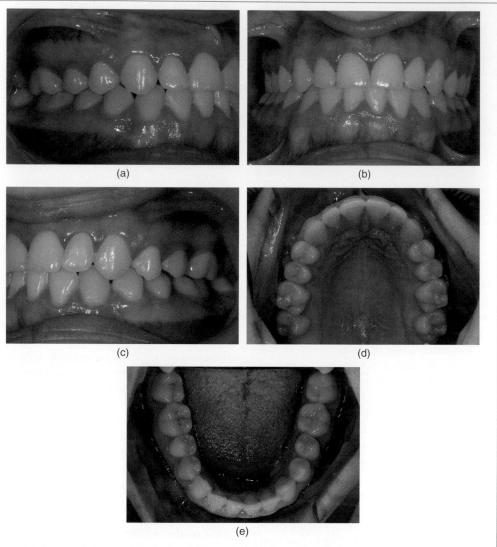

(a)

(b)

(c)

(d)

(e)

Figure 4.9 Intra oral photos: right, frontal, left occlusion (a–c), and occlusal view of the maxillary (d) and mandibular jaw (e).

a lateral head radiograph is useful when planning the orthodontic treatment; occasionally, the lateral head radiograph is indicated to be taken at different time intervals to monitor growth before and after treatment to evaluate treatment effects and from these findings decide the retention strategies. In addition, radiographs assessed within a patient on different occasions can be superimposed, thereby describing which changes have taken place during the interval between the radiographic exposures. The changes may express the treatment effects, growth or both. Many different analysable systems for lateral head radiographs

are available, which implies that no single system is satisfactory for all purposes and that all the systems have their advantages and disadvantages.

Finally, for research purposes after ethical approval, the lateral head radiograph can be a useful tool to obtain information on growth and development in longitudinal studies, but also for comparative studies considering treatment outcomes between new and established orthodontic methods.

In certain orthodontic cases, the 3D imaging like Cone Beam Computered Tomography (CBCT) may provide accurate information. Consequently, CBCT can be a valuable tool in

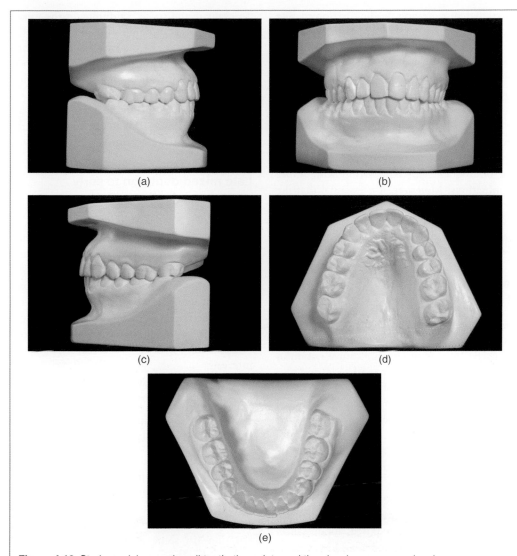

Figure 4.10 Study models covering all teeth, the palate and the alveolar processes (a–e).

the location of impacted teeth and resorption of adjacent teeth, assessment of alveolar bone height and volume and in the planning process of combined orthodontic and orthognathic surgery cases.

Important examinations at different dental developmental stages

The classifications of malocclusions in sagittal, vertical and transversal relation; dental crowding or spacing; and functional conditions shall always be registered. However, it can still be noted that even if a basic concept is followed when a patient is examined, it is important to remember to focus on specific tooth and occlusal anomalies and functional disturbances during the different physiological and psychological developmental stages that the patient undergoes.

The primary dentition (3–5 years of age)

At the primary dentition stage, an extra- and intra oral examination including the lips, cheeks and muscles is performed. The focus is on sucking habits and their consequences, eventual functional disturbances leading to forced bite and asymmetries of the face. In cases with anterior crossbite, it can be relevant to discuss the family history, since anterior crossbite may be an expression of genetic patterns.

In most children who show alterations or disturbances, there is as yet no indication for treatment, but the development of the alteration/disturbance should be followed. It is recommended to perform extra- and intra oral photographs for comparison with future examinations. Moreover, it is essential that the patient and the parents receive professional advice, which explains why treatment will be postponed.

Early mixed dentition (6–8 years of age)

During the early mixed dentition period, the dental and skeletal development is very pronounced. There is also a significant variation in development between boys and girls, and also within gender. Because of the large individual variations, it is important with regular annual check-ups to disclose expected and unexpected changes in development.

During this period, it is also advisable to be aware of asymmetrical tooth eruption patterns; this applies especially to the maxillary lateral incisor. If one lateral incisor has erupted and the contralateral is not visible within 3 to 6 months, further investigation is required, for instance, with an intra oral radiograph.

Focus is put on the following:

■ whether the maxillary first permanent molars are erupting normally;
■ whether the maxillary central incisors are in normal positions and whether there is a normal inter relation between maxillary and mandibular incisors;
■ whether the lateral incisors are present or if agenesis is suspected;
■ whether large overjet without sufficient lip closure is evident;
■ whether the mandible is guided laterally, creating a unilateral posterior crossbite, or whether the mandible is forced forwards and an anterior crossbite is established.

To evaluate the space conditions in the mixed dentition, a rule of thumb could be that the distance between the mesial surface of the first permanent molar and distal surface of the permanent lateral incisor should be at least 22 mm in the maxilla and 21 mm in the mandible.

When tooth and occlusal anomalies are discovered, it is advisable to consult or refer the patient to an orthodontist.

Late mixed dentition to early permanent dentition (9–12 years of age)

Also, at the late mixed dentition to early permanent dentition stage, a wide range of growth and dental and occlusal development is observed. Some children can be at the beginning of mixed dentition, while others of the same age have a fully formed permanent dentition. It is therefore essential to have appropriate examination intervals and rules with at least 1 year examination intervals.

At the beginning of this development stage, it is important to consider whether:

■ the maxillary canines are in normal positions;
■ the second premolars are present.

To disclose ectopically positioned canines, the alveolar process in the canine region should be palpated from both the buccal and palatal sides. Normally, a bulge appears in the buccal sulcus in the canine region 1 to 1.5 years before eruption (in some children at the age of 8 and at the latest at 10–11 years of age). If the canine cannot be palpated or there is an evident asymmetry between the contra lateral sides, there is reason to suspect an eruption disturbance, and a complementary radiographic investigation is indicated to disclose the position of the canine and evaluate the risk of root resorption on adjacent teeth.

To discover agenesis of the second premolar, previously taken bite-wing radiographs for caries diagnosis can be beneficial. If the premolar is not disclosed on those radiographs, periapical radiographs or a panoramic radiograph has to be assessed.

During this stage, it is also essential to try to find reasonable causes for the malocclusions.

For instance, if an anterior open bite is present, questions arise as to whether the open bite is caused by prolonged sucking habits or if hereditary factors are involved. In addition, if an anterior crossbite exists, hereditary factors are probably involved, and a genuine Class III malocclusion development may be expected later. Thus, for these patients, accurate registrations are valuable, often in the form of photos, study models and lateral head radiographs.

Early adolescence – permanent dentition (13–15 years of age)

As in previous dentition stages, it is important to examine and classify malocclusions in sagittal, vertical and transversal relation; dental crowding or spacing; and to register functional conditions. At the early adolescence to permanent dentition stage, it is also important to check that nothing in the previous stages has been missed, such as incorrect eruption of maxillary canines or agenesis of teeth.

Early adolescent patients presenting malocclusions and desire for orthodontic treatment will be referred, at this point, for specialist examination and evaluation for such treatment. Dental crowding or increased overjet are often the main problems for these patients.

Adolescence – permanent dentition (16–19 years of age)

Growth has now mostly ceased, and most malocclusions should have been treated before this age period. The exception is malocclusions with large skeletal discrepancies for which the treatment has consciously been postponed to await completion of growth. These severe malocclusions will be treated by combined orthodontic and orthognathic surgery treatment.

Adults

Generally, examination of adults is similar to examination of adolescents, but with some important additions.

For adult patients, the number and condition of the teeth can vary greatly, and pathological migration of teeth during the years may have caused functional disturbed occlusion and temporomandibular dysfunctions. It is also important and necessary to make a full periodontal examination for most of the adult patients. It must be noted that in patients who have periodontitis, the orthodontic treatment should be postponed until sufficient periodontal health has been achieved, and then the orthodontic treatment is assessed in cooperation with specialists in periodontology and/or dental hygienists.

There are several reasons why many adults demand orthodontic treatment. It may be that an adult did not previously have the opportunity to gain orthodontic treatment because there was no orthodontic care available. Other reasons include the relapse of a previous orthodontic treatment or that during orthodontic treatment at a younger age the patient failed to cooperate resulting in unsuccessful treatment results. Furthermore, the general demand for orthodontic care among adults has increased, because of the great emphasis put on appearance and aesthetics.

Like adolescent patients, adult patients want to correct discrepancies in the aesthetic area, for instance crowded incisors and spacing of teeth or missing teeth.

Conclusions

The results from the interview, clinical examination, extra- and intra oral photographs, as well as supplementary model and radiographic analyses, will constitute a solid basis for comprehensive orthodontic diagnosis, which in turn supports the treatment planning. Further on, before it is time to make a treatment plan, the dentist should ensure that the patient is motivated, psychologically prepared and informed about the advantages and disadvantages of treatment. For children and adolescents, it is also important that they have the support of their parents to complete the orthodontic treatment.

Later, when the treatment plan is presented, information is given regarding how the treatment goals will be reached, and then risks and requirements for the patient must be confirmed by the patient and the parents. Sometimes the agreement is signed in writing.

REFERENCES

Bondemark, L., Jeppsson, M., Lindh-Ingildsen, L. *et al.* (2006) Incidental findings of pathology and abnormality in pretreatment orthodontic panoramic radiographs. Angle Orthod 76: 98–102.

Dimberg, L., Lennartsson, B., Arnrup, K. *et al.* (2015) Prevalence and change of malocclusions from primary to early permanent dentition: a longitudinal study. Angle Orthod 85: 728–734.

List, T., Wahlund, K., Wenneberg, B. and Dworkin, S.F. (1999) TMD in children and adolescents: prevalence of pain, gender differences, and perceived treatment need. J Orofac Pain 13: 9–20.

Magnusson, T. and Helkimo, M. (2009) Temporomandibular disorders. In: *Pediatric Dentistry* (Eds G. Koch, and S. Poulsen) Blackwell Publishing Ltd, Oxford. pp. 310-311.

Nilsson, I.M., List, T. and Drangsholt, M. (2006) The reliability and validity of self-reported temporomandibular disorder pain in adolescents. J Orofac Pain 20: 138–144.

Petti, S. (2015) Over two hundred million injuries to anterior teeth attributable to large overjet: a meta-analysis. Dent Traumat 31: 1–8.

Schiffman, E., Ohrbach, R., Truelove, E. *et al.* (2014) International RDC/TMD Consortium Network, International association for Dental Research; Orofacial Pain Special Interest Group, International Association for the Study of Pain. Diagnostic Criteria for Temporomandibular Disorders (DC/TMD) for Clinical and Research Applications: recommendations of the International RDC/TMD Consortium Network* and Orofacial Pain Special Interest Group†. J Oral Facial Pain Headache 28: 6–27.

van der Linden, F.P.G.M. and Boersma, H. (1987) *Diagnosis and Treatment Planning in Dentofacial Orthopedics*. Quintessence Publishing Co, Ltd, Berlin. pp. 81–85.

PART 2

Treatment Principles of Skeletal and Dentoalveolar Anomalies

The differential diagnosis is of vital importance in therapy planning, and applies to discrepancy between the jaws (malocclusions in sagittal, vertical, transversal planes), as well as to anomalies within the jaws (crowding, spacing, single teeth).

The treatment outline, the optimal treatment period in the individual case, and finally suitable appliances will be discussed for the different anomalies.

Essential Orthodontics, First Edition. Birgit Thilander, Krister Bjerklin and Lars Bondemark.
© 2018 John Wiley & Sons Ltd. Published 2018 by John Wiley & Sons Ltd.

PART 2

Treatment Principles of Skeletal and Dentoalveolar Anomalies

CHAPTER 5

Sagittal, vertical and transversal discrepancies between the jaws

Lars Bondemark

Key topics

- Cephalometric analysis – differential diagnosis
- Treatment of Angle Class II malocclusions
- Treatment of Angle Class III malocclusions
- Treatment of deep bite
- Treatment of open bite
- Treatment of crossbite
- Treatment of scissors bite

Learning objectives

- To have an overview of how to carry out a cephalometric analysis
- To be able to make a differential diagnosis with respect to skeletal and dentoalveolar discrepancies
- To know how to treat different Angle Class II and III malocclusions
- To know how to treat deep and open bites
- To know how to treat crossbite and to understand the difference between slow and rapid expansion treatment
- To know how to treat scissors bite

Essential Orthodontics, First Edition. Birgit Thilander, Krister Bjerklin and Lars Bondemark.
© 2018 John Wiley & Sons Ltd. Published 2018 by John Wiley & Sons Ltd.

Introduction

To determine the sagittal and vertical positions of the jaws in relation to the cranial base and to classify the discrepancies that may exist between the jaws, it is important to make a differential diagnosis. In order to fully evaluate the proportion of skeletal discrepancy, a lateral head radiograph together with a cephalometric analysis is a valuable tool to assess and then be used together with the clinical evaluation to create a complete diagnosis. Consequently, to assess an accurate differential diagnosis with respect to skeletal and dentoalveolar discrepancies, a cephalometric analysis is needed.

Cephalometric analysis

A cephalometric analysis is performed on a lateral head radiograph. The lateral head radiograph exposure is assessed with the patient's head standardised oriented in a cephalostat. The cephalostat has ear rods to set the patient so that the midsagittal plane of the head will be parallel to the film plane at a fixed distance from the X-ray tube. The head should be positioned according to the Frankfurt horizontal, or in a natural head posture, and the teeth shall be in central occlusion.

The main objectives with a cephalometric analysis is to classify the facial type, show the skeletal jaw conditions in relation to the cranial base, and thereby provide a basis to assess an accurate differential diagnosis with respect to skeletal and dentoalveolar discrepancies. Furthermore, it is possible to evaluate growth or treatment results by making cephalometric analyses at different time intervals.

To assimilate and carry out a cephalometric analysis, it is important to have a good knowledge of hard and soft tissue anatomy, since the analysis is based on measurements on and between well-defined anatomical bony points and contours.

There exist different cephalometric analyses, and they can be categorised roughly into two types. One type is described as evaluation of the patient by means of specific ideal values that are applied to assign the treatment objective, and thus the analysis leads to the definition of the treatment itself. Steiner and Tweed's analyses are examples of such analyses. The other type, demonstrated by Björk (1955), is designed to discern whether malocclusions are of dentoalveolar or skeletal origin, or the role of the interaction between the sagittal and vertical development and its impact on the craniofacial skeleton.

It can be pointed out that cephalometric values vary between ethnic groups but also between gender and age (Thilander *et al.*, 2005); thus, awareness that cephalometric standards may differ between groups is of importance for orthodontic diagnosis and treatment planning.

Björk's analysis will be briefly illustrated, and the cephalometric values for this analysis described below are representative of a Scandinavian population. Figures 5.1 and 5.2 show some key reference points and lines used for the cephalometric analysis according to Björk, aside from the points 'ss' and 'sm' defined as 'A' and 'B', respectively.

With help of the analysis, it can be determined whether an individual has a sagittal relationship with a normal maxillary position and a retrognathic mandible, a prognathic maxilla

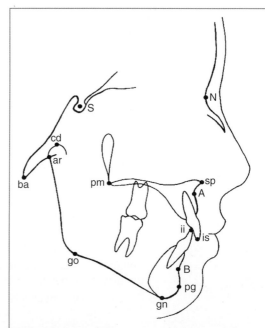

Figure 5.1 Examples of reference points used in the cephalometric analysis according to Björk (1955).

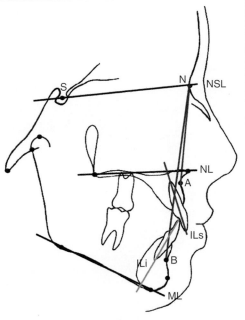

Figure 5.2 Important reference lines and angles according to Björk (1955). Lines: NSL = cranial base line; NL = nasal line; ML = mandibular line. Angles: SNA = sagittal relation of the maxilla; SNB = sagittal relation of the mandible; ANB = sagittal inter jaw relation; ILs/NL maxillary incisor inclination; Ili/ML = mandibular incisor inclination; NSL/NL = vertical inclination of the maxilla; NSL/ML = vertical inclination of the mandible; NL/ML = vertical inter jaw relation.

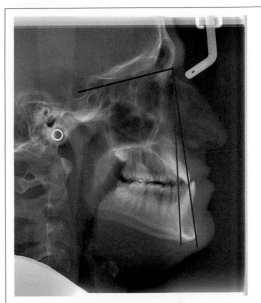

Figure 5.3 Class III skeletal relation, i.e. a negative ANB angle implying the SNA angle (the angle between the black and blue line) is smaller than the SNB angle (the angle between the black and red line).

and a normal mandibular position, or combinations of maxillary and mandibular prognathism and retrognathism. Consequently, by using the nasion sella line (NSL, equivalent to the cranial base), the sagittal relation of the maxilla (SNA angle) and the mandible (SNB angle) in relation to the cranial base can be determined as well as the interrelation between the maxilla and mandible (ANB angle). Even if the values of the different cephalometric variables differ depending on age and ethnicity, the normal value for a Scandinavian population is 82° ± 3.5° for SNA, SNB 79° ± 3.5° and for ANB 3° ± 2.5°. In a case with a negative ANB angle (skeletal Class III relation) (Figure 5.3), this can be explained by either a normal SNA and a large SNB angle (mandibular prognathism) or a small SNA (maxillary retrognathism) and a normal SNB angle. On the other hand, if a large

ANB angle is evident (skeletal Class II relation) (Figure 5.4), it may be due to either a normal SNA and a small SNB angle (mandibular retrognathism) or a great SNA (maxillary prognathism) and a normal SNB angle. Of course, there may also exist combinations of the relations or conditions described above.

Regarding the vertical relation, the nasal line (NL or sp-pm, Figures 5.1 and 5.2) and mandibular line (ML, Figure 5.2) are designed lines where NLs match that of the nasal floor and the upper part of the maxilla (equivalent to the vertical inclination of the maxilla), and ML corresponds to the mandibular lower border (equivalent to the vertical inclination of the mandible). The angle between the NSL and ML, as well as the NSL and NL, measures the face height. The normal value for NSL/ML is 33° ± 6° and for NSL/NL 8° ± 3.0°. If a low-angle, mandible plan related to the cranial base is evident (NSL/ML<27°, hypodivergent or low-angle), this implies a skeletal deep overbite accompanied by an upward and forward growth rotation of the mandible (Figure 5.5). In a vertically opposite relationship, that is, at

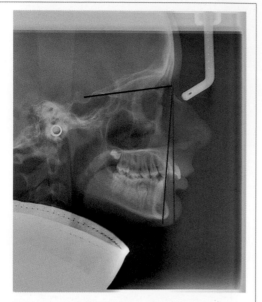

Figure 5.4 Class II skeletal relation, i.e. a positive ANB angle implying the SNA angle (black and blue line) is larger (>5 degrees) than the SNB angle (black and red line).

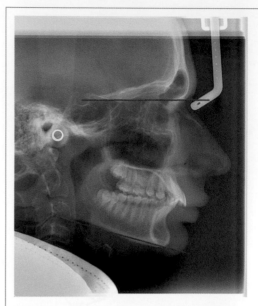

Figure 5.5 Low-angle or hypodivergent case, the angle between NSL and ML is small implying a skeletal deep overbite.

a high-angle mandibular plane related to the cranial base (NSL/ML > 39°, hyperdivergent or high-angle), an increased anterior face height exists associated by a backward and posterior growth rotation of the mandible (Figure 5.6).

Finally, the maxillary and mandibular incisor inclinations are determined. A normal maxillary incisor inclination (ILs/NL) is 110° ± 6°, and the normal mandibular incisor inclination (ILi/ML) is 94° ± 7°. If the angle is greater than normal, the incisors are proclined, and the incisors are retroclined if a smaller inclination than normal exists.

Thus, the sagittal, vertical and incisor inclination deviations obtained for a certain patient can be used for determination of whether the observed difference in occlusion is of dental or skeletal origin.

When treatment results are evaluated, it is necessary to take at least two lateral head radiographs, one before and one at the end of treatment. The purpose is to describe what changes have taken place during the time

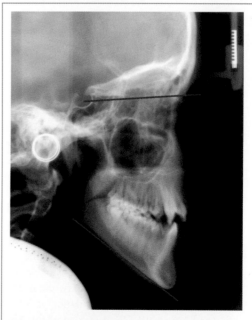

Figure 5.6 High-angle or hyperdivergent case, the angle between NSL and ML is large implying a skeletal open bite.

interval between the exposures. Accordingly, the two lateral head radiographs should be superimpositioned on stable structures of the cranial base. It is well known that the anterior part, or wall, of the sella turcica is stable, as well as the anterior portion of the cranial base, and does not change in connection with growth after the age of 7 years (see also Chapter 3). Consequently, by superimposition of the two radiographs on the stable structures, the amount of treatment effects can be evaluated.

Treatment of Angle Class II malocclusion

Angle Class II malocclusion (postnormal occlusion) is a common malocclusion, with a frequency between 14 and 18%. The main treatment goals are to create normal molar and incisor relations with a well-disposed inter-jaw sagittal and vertical morphology. Another treatment goal is to achieve normal lip closure and thereby reduce the trauma risk of the maxillary incisors (Thiruvenkatachari et al., 2013), and to prevent children from being teased or bullied (de Oliveira and Sheiham, 2003) for their proclined and visible maxillary incisors (see Figure 4.3 in Chapter 4).

Many treatment options are available for correction of Angle Class II malocclusions depending on what part of the craniofacial skeleton is affected. Consequently, in therapy planning of Class II malocclusion cases, a differential diagnosis of sagittal and vertical jaw relations as well as incisor positions must be performed.

Angle Class II division 1 malocclusion

The typical patient with Angle Class II division 1 occlusion often has an increased overjet, incomplete lip closure, deep bite, mandibular retrognathism and a convex profile. Class II division 1 treatment is normally accomplished in two phases: first the inter-jaw discrepancies are corrected by orthopaedic forces; subsequently, a second treatment phase is started to create optimal Class I occlusion and alignment of teeth.

Treatment in mixed dentition

A functional appliance producing orthopaedic forces can be used. The Andrésen activator (Andrésen et al., 1957), one of the first functional appliances that attained extensive clinical use, is constructed to alter the functional pattern and simultaneously stimulate muscle activity that is converted to forces designed to move the teeth in all three planes of space. Thus, the mandible is moved forwards for correction of the Class II malocclusion and opens the bite. In addition, a retroclination of maxillary incisors and proclination of mandibular incisors will be created to promote normal lip closure (Figure 5.7a–c).

It is often necessary to start the treatment with a transversal expansion of the maxilla to achieve appropriate width for the maxilla when the mandible is in the advanced position.

Other functional appliances for Angle Class II malocclusion correction are the Harvold activator (Vargervik and Harvold, 1985), Frankel function regulator (Freeman et al., 2009), Bass appliance (Bass, 1982) and Clark's twin-block (Clark, 2010). Functional appliances can also be combined with headgear, the aim of which is to restrain the forward growth of the maxilla (Figure 5.7d). There are several types of headgear activators, and some common ones are the van Beek activator (van Beek, 1982) and Zürich activator (Teuscher, 1987).

Treatment in early adolescence

The treatment choice depends on the dentoalveolar and skeletal situation. In cases with Class II division 1 malocclusion, mandibular retrognathism and deep bite, a fixed appliance in both jaws combined with Class II elastics can be used. The Class II elastics support the correction of Class II malocclusion and open the bite (Figure 5.8). However, if the co-operation with the Class II elastics is judged to fail, a Forsus spring can be inserted (Heinig and Göz, 2001). The Forsus spring is a Herbst appliance hybrid, non-removable by the patients and with a flexible connection between the maxillary molar headgear tube and the mandibular archwire, creating a mesial force on the mandibular and a

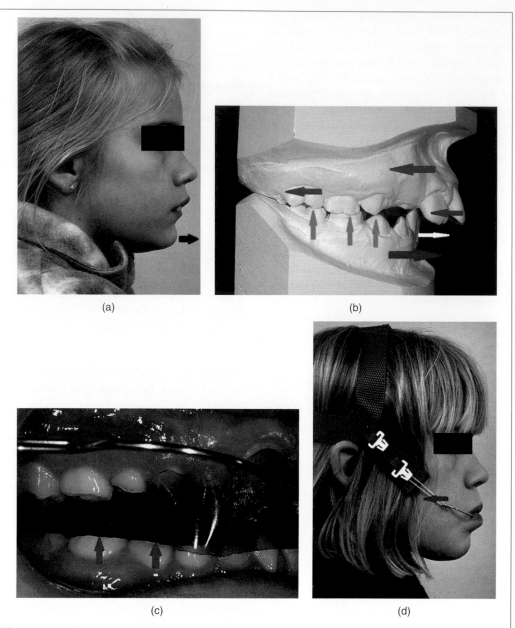

(a)

(b)

(c)

(d)

Figure 5.7 In this case the intention is with a functional appliance to move the mandible forward (a) for correction of the Class II malocclusion and simultaneously opens the bite as well as retroclination of the maxillary incisors (blue arrow) and proclination of mandibular incisors (white arrow in b). In (c), the occlusal acrylic over the mandibular molars and premolars has been removed to allow those teeth to vertically over-erupt (blue arrows), and thereby create bite opening. The functional appliances can also be combined with a headgear (d) to restrain the forward growth of the maxilla (red arrow).

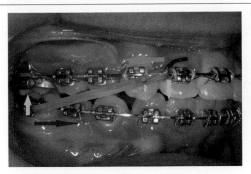

Figure 5.8 Class II elastics for correction of a Class II malocclusion. The objective is to create a Class I occlusion by distal movement of the maxillary teeth (green arrow) and mesial movement of the corresponding mandibular teeth (red arrow). The force distribution of Class II elastics also results in a bite opening effect (yellow arrows).

distal force on the maxillary arch. In even more severe Class II division 1 malocclusion cases with mandibular retrognathism, the Herbst appliance may be very useful. This appliance has been extensively described and evaluated (Pancherz and Ruf, 2008) (Figure 5.9). According to existing evidence, fixed functional appliances are effective in the short term to improve Class II malocclusion, but the effect is mainly dentoalveolar rather than skeletal (Zymperdikas *et al.*, 2016). Even if the evidence level of most included studies considering the Herbst appliance is rather low, good dento-skeletal stability without clinically relevant changes was found for most variables (Bock *et al.*, 2016).

If proclined maxillary incisors are evident because of mesial drift of the lateral segments and with normal skeletal relationship between the jaws, extraction of two maxillary premolars and fixed appliances in both jaws can correct the increased overjet and establish a stable occlusion with Class I relation between the canines and Class II relation between the molars (Figure 5.10).

Treatment of adults

In adults with severe mandibular deficiency/ retrognathism, combined orthodontic and surgical correction is recommended. A common orthognathic surgery procedure for setting forward the mandible is the sagittal split. In surgery cases, the risks of surgery should be within acceptable levels, and the benefits of surgical treatment should be obvious. However, some adult patients refuse combined orthodontic and surgical correction. Instead, a non-surgical correction of the Class II malocclusion is performed by dental camouflage to mask the skeletal discrepancy. The correction consists of bilateral extraction of maxillary premolars to give the possibilities to retract and retrocline the maxillary anterior dentition to achieve acceptable overjet and improved smile aesthetics. Even if the camouflage treatment is a compromise treatment, satisfactory results can be achieved with a functional occlusion and acceptable facial profile.

Angle Class II division 2 malocclusion

Treatment can be undertaken either in the mixed or in the permanent dentition. Since the malocclusion is associated with retroclined maxillary central incisors and often at least one proclined lateral incisor and deep bite, the treatment is usually achieved in three phases. The treatment starts with proclination of the incisors, i.e. the Class II division 2 malocclusion is converted to a Class II division 1 malocclusion. The proclination can be performed either with palatal springs in a removable appliance, or the incisors can be upright in a full-fixed appliance. In the second phase, the mandible is advanced and bite opening performed by a removable or fixed functional appliance. Finally, in the third phase, a multibracket fixed appliance is inserted in both jaws in combination with Class II elastics to create an optimal Class I occlusion and alignment of teeth.

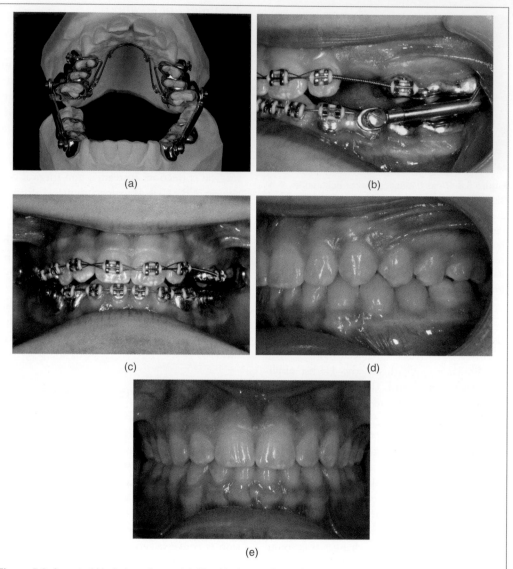

Figure 5.9 A casted Herbst appliance (a). The Herbst appliance in place with a forward movement of the mandible to an almost incisal edge-to-edge relation (b,c). A firm Class I occlusion result after treatment (d,e).

In severe skeletal Class II division 2 malocclusion cases in adults, treatment will start by orthodontic proclination of the maxillary incisors, and will often be similar to treatment of severe cases of Class II division 1, i.e. a combined orthodontic and surgical correction.

Treatment of Angle Class III malocclusion

The frequency of Angle Class III (prenormal occlusion) varies from 2.2 to 12%, depending on the ethnic group, age of the children studied and if an edge-to-edge relationship is included in the data. Higher frequencies of Class III malocclusions are reported in Asian populations (Ngan *et al.*, 1997). The condition may be dental or skeletal in origin. It may also be due to a functional, protrusive shift of the mandible caused by interference with the normal path of mandibular closure. This condition is referred to as pseudo Class III malocclusion or anterior crossbite with functional shift, and these are

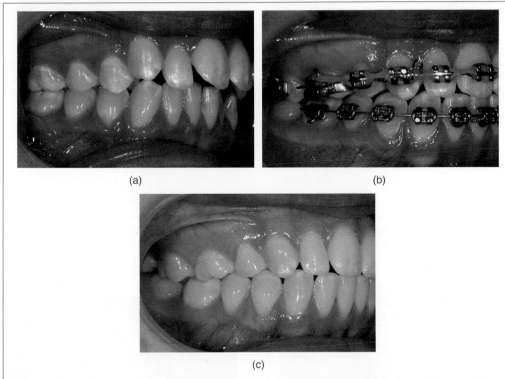

(a)

(b)

(c)

Figure 5.10 In this Class II malocclusion case with normal skeletal relationship between the jaws (a), bilateral extraction of the maxillary first premolars has been performed and then a fixed appliance in both jaws was inserted (b). The final treatment result (c) with a Class I relation between the canines and Class II relation between the molars.

skeletal Class I malocclusions (Thilander and Myrberg, 1973).

Cephalometrically, a skeletal Class III relationship is defined as a negative ANB angle. A skeletal Class III may be caused by either retrusion of the maxilla or protrusion of the mandible, or a combination of both. Moreover, skeletal Class III malocclusions are associated with various clefts in the maxilla as well as syndromes such as Apert and Cruzon.

Angle Class III with dental origin

Treatment in mixed dentition

Various treatment options are available for Class III malocclusions of dental origin, i.e. pseudo Class III or anterior crossbite with functional shift. In the mixed dentition, a common method is to use a removable appliance. The appliance consists of an acrylic plate with protruding springs or protruding screws for the maxillary incisors, with or without bilateral occlusal coverage of the posterior teeth (Figure 5.11). An additional labial bow for the mandibular incisors may also be incorporated into the acrylic plate in order to retrocline the mandibular incisors and to make it more difficult for the patient to achieve anterior shift of the mandible during treatment.

A fixed appliance can also be used (Figure 5.12) and consists of varying numbers of brackets and wires of different dimensions and materials, sometimes with loops and bends. Another variant is a so-called 2 × 4 appliance, comprising bands on the maxillary first permanent molars and brackets on the four maxillary incisors. A flexible wire is often used for nivellation, and a steel wire with advancing loops is used for proclination of the maxillary incisors (Rabie and Gu, 1999).

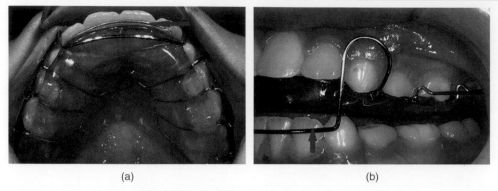

(a)   (b)

Figure 5.11 In (a), a removable appliance for correction of a Class III malocclusion (pseudo Class III) with a protrusion spring for proclination of the maxillary incisors (blue arrow). In (b), bilateral occlusal coverage (red arrow) of the maxillary posterior teeth to avoid vertical interlock between the incisors in crossbite. To retrocline the mandibular incisors, a labial bow has been inserted (blue arrow).

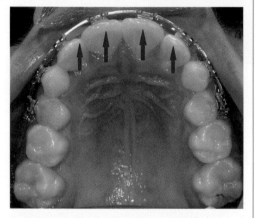

Figure 5.12 Fixed multibracket appliance for proclination of the maxillary incisors (red arrows) in a pseudo Class III malocclusion case.

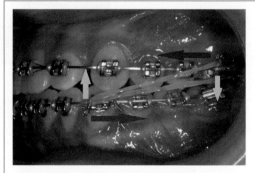

Figure 5.13 Class III elastics for correction of a Class III malocclusion. The objective is to create a Class I occlusion by mesial movement of the maxillary teeth (red arrow) and distal movement of the corresponding mandibular teeth (blue arrow). The force distribution of Class III elastics also results in a bite opening effect (yellow arrows).

A series of studies considering comparison of treatment with fixed and removable appliance for early orthodontic correction of pseudo Class III malocclusion has been performed (Wiedel, 2015). It was concluded that both removable and fixed appliances presented high success rates, demonstrated good long-term stability and were well accepted by the patients. However, treatment by removable appliance was the more expensive alternative, and therefore fixed appliances emerged as the preferred approach to correction of pseudo Class III malocclusion in mixed dentition.

Treatment in early adolescence

In permanent dentition, fixed appliances with Class III elastics can be used. Often, the elastics are hooked between the maxillary molar teeth and the mandibular anterior teeth, resulting in an anterior pull on the maxilla and distal pull on the mandible (Figure 5.13). If crowding is also evident, the treatment can be combined with extractions of the first mandibular premolars and second maxillary premolars, but this only permits mild Class III discrepancy to be camouflaged by tooth movements.

Angle Class III with skeletal origin

Treatment in mixed dentition

In Class III malocclusion subjects with mandibular prognathism, the treatment aims to restrain the mandibular forward growth or keep the mandible backwards with orthopaedic forces. On the other hand, in Class III cases with a retrognathic maxilla, orthopaedic forces can act on the maxillary sutures by enhancing the maxilla into a forward position.

Different kinds of extra-oral pull have been used to inhibit mandibular anterior growth and/or to enhance maxillary anterior growth. If the patient has a retrognathic maxilla, a protraction facemask, also called reverse headgear, can be used in mixed dentition (Delaire, 1997). The reverse headgear is applied to a fixed appliance in the maxilla by elastics pulling the maxilla forwards; pillows in the masks are applied to the forehead and chin, exerting a retrusive pull on the mandible at the same time (Figure 5.14). The reverse headgear is often combined with lateral expansion. In a multicentre randomised controlled trial of early Class III orthopaedic treatment with a protraction facemask and untreated controls, successful outcomes of Class I occlusions were reported in 70% of the subjects (Mandall et al., 2010).

Treatment in early adolescence

Bone-anchored miniplates have been used to treat Angle Class III malocclusion with maxillary retrusion (De Clerck and Swennen, 2011). The bilateral maxillary miniplate is fixed by three monocortical screws at the infrazygomatic crest and the bilateral mandibular miniplate with two screws between the lateral incisor and the canine. Class III elastics are inserted between the maxillary and mandibular miniplates to apply a protrusive force to the maxilla and a retrusive force to the mandible.

Treatment of adults

In adult cases of severe skeletal Class III malocclusions, the predominant recommended treatment method is a combination of bimaxillary fixed appliance and orthognathic surgery in the maxilla and/or mandible. The most common orthognathic surgery procedure in the maxilla is forward movement with Le Fort 1 osteotomy and in the mandible, either sagittal split or ramus osteotomy is used to set back the mandible.

Treatment prognosis

Factors reported to influence successful treatment of Angle Class III malocclusion include the age at which the appliance is inserted, the severity of the malocclusion, and heredity. Furthermore, if the patient can achieve an edge-to-edge incisor position, it may improve the prognosis for orthodontic correction. Less favourable factors for orthodontic treatment alone include mandibular prognathism with large negative ANB angle, large gonion angle, small cranial base angle and retroclined mandibular incisors (Thilander, 1965).

Long-term stability, especially for early treatment of Class III malocclusions of skeletal origin can be difficult to predict. In many cases, early treatment may be successful, and normal occlusion can be achieved. However, it should be remembered that the mandibular growth continues after maxillary growth has ceased, which implies an obvious risk for relapse of a previously corrected Class III malocclusion.

Treatment of deep bite

The frequency of deep bite is 8 to 11%, and this malocclusion often occurs along with Angle Class II malocclusions.

The purpose of treating deep bite is to reduce the overbite by incisor intrusion and proclination or extrusion of the molars or a combination of these methods. It is especially important to treat a deep bite if the overbite is so severe that the mandibular incisors impinge upon the palatal tissues behind the maxillary incisors.

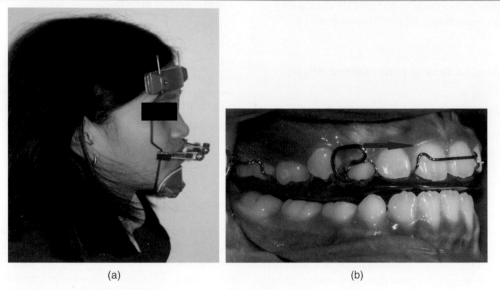

(a)   (b)

Figure 5.14 The reverse headgear (a) will be applied with elastics to a removable appliance in the maxilla (b) and move the jaw and teeth in a mesial direction (red arrow).

It is important to distinguish dentoalveolar from skeletal deep bite. The dentoalveolar deep bite is often caused by overeruption of incisors, lack of eruption of the lateral tooth segments or loss of molar support due to molar extractions. The skeletal deep bite shows a low-angle (hypodivergent) vertical mandible plan related to the cranial base (Figure 5.5), which implies a short anterior face height accompanied by an upward and forward growth rotation of the mandible.

Treatment in mixed dentition

An alternative to treating a deep bite in mixed dentition is to insert functional appliances, especially if the deep bite is combined with Angle Class II malocclusion. The use of a functional appliance allows the premolars and molars to vertically erupt while the incisors are held in place vertically or proclined (Figure 5.7b and c).

Treatment in early adolescence

For deep bite correction in the early adolescence, multibracket appliances in both jaws must be inserted to intrude the incisors and/or extrude the molars and premolars. Often, a reverse curve of Spee of the archwire is accomplished to produce a maximum bite opening effect, and it is recommended to engage the second molars into the multibracket appliance.

If the deep bite is extensive, bite opening can be facilitated by a fixed maxillary palatal biteplane. The biteplane is in occlusion with the mandibular incisors and canines, creating a separation space of 3 to 4 mm between the maxillary and mandibular molars (Figure 5.15). Bite opening could thereby be achieved by vertical overeruption of premolars and molars (Bondemark et al., 1994).

Treatment of open bite

In primary dentition, it is reported that 50% of 3-year-old children have anterior open bite. However, a large amount of these open bites self-correct as sucking habits cease, and thus, about 4% of school children and adolescents show open bite.

Morphologically, open bite can be categorised as being of dentoalveolar or skeletal origin. The dentoalveolar open bite is usually caused by impaired eruption of anterior maxillary or mandibular teeth together with deficient vertical development of the alveolar process.

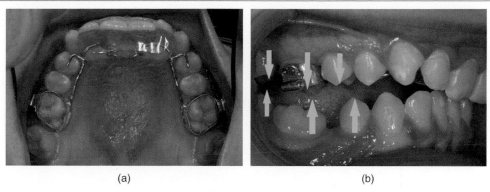

(a)   (b)

Figure 5.15 A fixed bite plane cemented with bands on the first maxillary molars (a). In occlusion, the mandibular incisors are in contact with the bite plane and between the maxillary and mandibular premolars and molars, a separation space of 3 to 4 mm is created (b), for vertical development of the lateral segments (yellow arrows) and thereby bite opening.

In skeletal open bite, a high-angle (hyperdivergent) mandibular plane related to the cranial base is evident, implying an increased anterior face height that is associated by a backward or posterior growth rotation of the mandible (Figure 5.6). In skeletal open bite cases, the prognosis for stable treatment results is highly dependent on the remaining growth. Therefore, the treatment is often postponed until the growth has terminated.

The skeletal open bite is mostly of hereditary origin, but environmental factors can contribute to open bite, among them are sucking habits, tongue thrust and breathing deficiency due to obstructive pharyngeal airways. The obstructions may be caused by large adenoids and tonsils or swollen mucosa due to allergies. In addition, changes in muscle function associated with an extended head posture as well as prolonged obstruction of nose breathing can contribute to the further development of a skeletal open bite.

Treatment in primary and mixed dentition

Treatment is often based on functional and aesthetic reasons. In primary and early mixed dentition, the focus is on breaking the sucking habits. If the sucking habits terminate at 6 to 7 years of age, the prospect is good for self-correction of the open bite. On the other hand, if the sucking habit has not terminated by this age and the child is psychologically motivated for treatment, treatment can be accomplished with a lingual arch or removable acrylic plate with a crib. The crib will prevent the child from sucking the finger or thumb, as well as prevent the tongue being forced in between the maxillary and mandibular incisors during swallowing (Figure 5.16). The crib may be perceived as bulky or uncomfortable, but it is remarkably well tolerated by most children. If the appliance contributes to breaking the sucking habit, it is advisable to continue the treatment for a further half a year to prevent relapse of the habit. However, if the sucking habit still does not cease despite treatment, it may be appropriate in these rare cases to refer the child to a child psychologist for evaluation of whether the habit is symptom of a psychological disturbance.

When respiratory obstruction is evident and suspected to be the cause of the open bite, an ear, nose and throat specialist should be consulted to consider whether, for example, large adenoids or tonsils are apparent, and if so, whether adenoidectomy or tonsillectomy is recommended to remove the respiratory obstruction.

Treatment in early adolescence

A dentoalveolar open bite can be treated with intrusion of premolars and molars with lateral bite splints. Another alternative is to use a

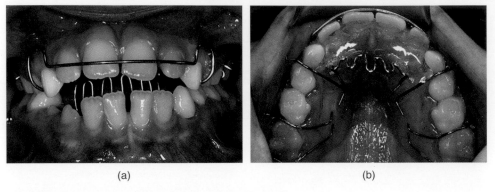

(a)   (b)

Figure 5.16 In (a,b), a removable appliance with a vertical crib.

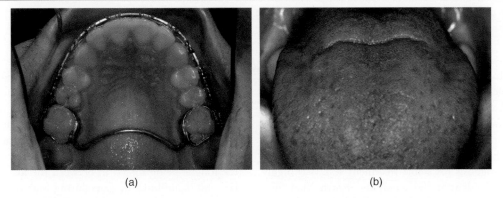

(a)   (b)

Figure 5.17 A transpalatal bar soldered to the maxillary first molar bands (a). Since the bar is 6 to 8 mm away from the palatal mucosa, there will be pressure by the tongue on the bar and this pressure causes intrusion forces on the maxillary first molars. A clear imprint by the bar can be seen on the tongue (b), indicating pressure by the bar on the tongue.

transpalatal bar soldered to bands of the maxillary first molars. There shall be a 6 to 8 mm space between the bar and the palatal mucosa, allowing for intrusion of the molars by pressure of the tongue when swallowing (Figure 5.17). The intrusion effect can also be further increased if a high-pull headgear is combined with the transpalatal bar. The treatment will then be completed by multibracket appliances to carefully align and extrude the incisors with light vertical intermaxillary elastics, with or without multi-loop archwires. It must be remembered that intrusion of molars and premolars with conventional orthodontics, as described above, is a difficult task. Therefore, insertion of mini implants or miniscrews for skeletal anchorage can be very useful when molars and premolars are intruded (Hart *et al.*, 2015).

Treatment of adults

Regardless of the treatment method used for correcting skeletal open bite, the prognosis for stable treatment results is highly dependent on the remaining growth. Consequently, to await the completion of growth is very important in cases of severe skeletal open bites, i.e. high-angle or long-face cases. In such cases, the patient will be treated with a combination of a bimaxillary fixed orthodontic appliance and orthognathic surgery.

Treatment of posterior crossbite

The frequency of posterior crossbite is reported to be 8.5 to 17%, and the wide range of frequency can be attributed to lack of uniformity in the different studies with respect to subject age, population, sample size and definitions. The majority of posterior crossbites are unilateral and are of three types:

1 due to disproportion between the jaws in skeletal width;
2 discrepancy in dentoalveolar width; and
3 associated with a forced guidance of the mandible, deviating the midline of the mandible to the crossbite side (Figure 2.9 in Chapter 2).

A bilateral crossbite is caused by a transversal skeletal constriction of the maxilla (crossbite of skeletal origin) without a forced guidance of the mandible.

Self-correction of a unilateral posterior crossbite can occur (Thilander *et al.*, 1984), but the rates of self-correction and development of new malocclusions has shown to be similar between 3 and 7 years of age (Dimberg *et al.*, 2013). If a sucking habit is discontinued early, the conditions for self-correction are favourable, since the tongue position and muscular activity can be normalised. Moreover, differences between intercanine and intermolar widths in the maxilla and mandible can be of importance for self-correction as well as when treatment with an expansion appliance is inserted. Thus, a narrow crossbite side in the maxillary arch together with a broad crossbite side in the mandible will result in a higher amount of non-correction cases (Thilander and Lennartsson, 2002).

Treatment in primary dentition

Cases of moderate transverse discrepancies may be treated in the primary dentition by grinding the interfering cusps of the deciduous teeth (Thilander *et al.*, 1984). The main aim with grinding is to eliminate the premature contacts causing the deviation of the mandible. To succeed with the grinding treatment, the maxillary arch width should be at least 3 mm greater in the canine region than the corresponding mandibular arch width. If the maxillary arch is narrower, treatment shall be performed in the mixed dentition by an orthodontic appliance to expand the maxilla.

Treatment in mixed dentition

Expansion

Treatment with maxillary expansion can be achieved rapidly, in 2 to 3 weeks, using a rapid maxillary expansion (RME) appliance. For RME, orthopaedic forces deliver expansion of the median palatal suture.

Expansion may also be gradual or slow (3–14 months) using, for example, a Quad Helix appliance or an expansion plate. The difference in expansion rates reflects differences in the frequencies of activation, the magnitude of applied force, the duration of treatment and the proportion of dentoalveolar to skeletal effects.

Slow expansion

The Quad Helix is a fixed appliance comprising stainless steel bands cemented onto the maxillary first molars and a standard stainless steel arch attached to the palatal surfaces of the teeth (Figure 5.18). Once inserted, the appliance is not dependent on patient compliance. The expansion of the steel arch (normally 10 mm before insertion) exerts a lateral force on the teeth, resulting in a predominant transverse dentoalveolar expansion of the maxillary arch. If necessary, the appliance can be reactivated after 6 weeks.

Also, a removable maxillary appliance can be used. The appliance consists of an acrylic

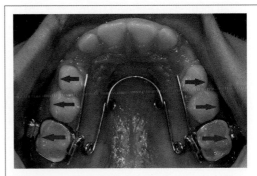

Figure 5.18 A Quad Helix. When the Quad Helix is inserted, the lingual arch with the 4 loops are transversally compressed, resulting in expansion forces on the teeth (blue arrows).

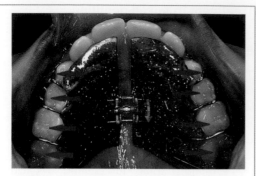

Figure 5.19 A removable acrylic expansion plate is retained with clasps on the maxillary first permanent molars and the deciduous first molars. The screw in the middle of the plate is activated once or twice a week (0.2–0.4 mm), producing transversal expansion forces on the teeth (red arrows).

palatal plate with a central expansion screw, retained by stainless steel clasps on the first primary and permanent molars (Figure 5.19). To expand the plate, the screw is activated one or two notches per week (0.2–0.4 mm), exerting pressure on the teeth in contact with the plate, thus mostly dentoalveolar expansion is created. The appliance is intended to be worn day and night, except for meals and tooth brushing, and thus is highly dependent on patient compliance.

For correction of unilateral posterior crossbite in mixed dentition, it has been proved that the Quad Helix appliance is superior to the expansion plate in terms of effectiveness and cost-minimisation and is therefore the preferred method of treatment (Petrén *et al.*, 2013). However, if the treatment with an expansion plate has been successful, this method shows similar long-term stability to treatment with the Quad Helix (Bjerklin, 2000; Petrén *et al.*, 2011).

When a single molar or premolar is in crossbite, a cross-elastic pull can be used (Figure 5.20). The elastic pull provides a reciprocal force, i.e. buccal-occlusal action on the maxillary molar or premolar and a lingual-occlusal action on the mandibular molar or premolar. The prognosis for cross-elastic treatment relies on patient co-operation and whether a firm cuspal interlocking has been created after the correction.

Rapid expansion

When RME is carried out, orthopaedic forces create expansion of the maxillary median palatal suture (Figure 5.21), but dentoalveolar expansion effects are also produced. The suture expansion is around 20 to 50% of the total screw expansion (Bazargani *et al.*, 2013). It should be pointed out that RME also leads to an increased dimension of the nasal cavity (Ballanti *et al.*, 2010) and moderate evidence exists that RME in growing children improves the conditions for nasal breathing from a short-term perspective (Baratieri *et al.*, 2011).

RME is performed using a fixed appliance. The Haas and Hyrax appliances are the most common, and the main difference between these appliances is that the Haas appliance has tooth and palatal mucosa supported anchorage (Figure 5.22), while the Hyrax appliance only has tooth supported anchorage, comprising stainless steel bands cemented onto the maxillary first molars and premolars and a standard stainless steel arch attached to a palatal screw (Figure 5.21). The screw is activated once or twice a day, normally 0.2 mm per activation, and both appliances have been shown to be effective in correcting transverse maxillary deficiency (Weissheimer *et al.*, 2011). Moreover, temporary anchorage devices (TADs) can be used as skeletal anchorage in combination with the expansion appliance. Thus, miniscrews can be inserted on each side of the median palatal suture to replace teeth as anchorage units (Ludwig *et al.*, 2013).

RME can also be successfully achieved for unilateral or bilateral posterior crossbite without engaging the permanent teeth (Cozzani *et al.*, 2007). A modified Haas-type RME appliance is used, and the appliance is anchored to the maxillary primary molars and canines (Figure 5.22). Consequently, no forces are placed on the permanent molars; nevertheless, there will be an increase in intermolar width between the permanent molars, and the expansion has also been found to be stable at least 2 years after intervention (Cozzani *et al.*, 2007).

In severe maxillary transverse constriction or after growth has ceased, orthodontic treatment alone is not sufficient for successful expansion. These cases require a combination of surgery and

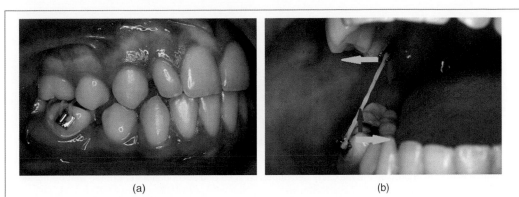

Figure 5.20 In (a), a cross-elastic between a palatal placed bracket on the right maxillary first molar and a buccal bracket on the right mandibular first molar. In (b), the maxillary molar is moved buccally and the mandibular molar lingually (yellow arrows). Both molars are also extruded (red arrows).

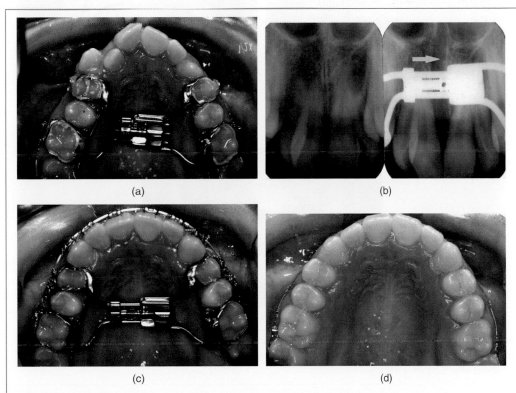

Figure 5.21 A RME appliance cemented on the maxillary first premolars and molars (a). The central screw is activated once or twice a day corresponding to an expansion of between 0.2 and 0.4 mm. Intra oral radiographs of maxillary incisors before and after RME (b,c). The X-ray image (c) shows a clear widening of the median palatal suture (yellow arrow). After expansion, a multibracket fixed appliance has created good alignment of the teeth (d), and the result after 1.5 years of treatment (e).

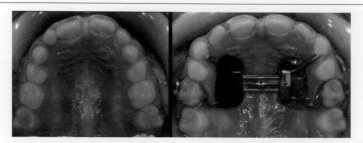

Figure 5.22 A modified Haas-type RME appliance for expansion in the early mixed dentition. Note that the appliance is only anchored on the maxillary deciduous canines and second molars. Photos with permission of Dr Marco Rosa, Italy.

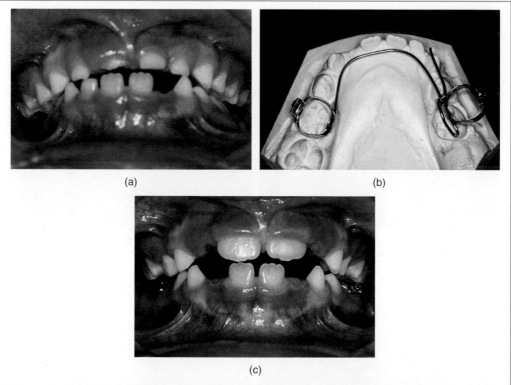

Figure 5.23 A bilateral completely scissors bite (a). A fixed lingual arch with bands on mandibular first molars for transversal expansion of the mandibular arch (b). Transversal expansion of the mandibular arch achieved after 5 months' treatment (c).

orthodontic treatment, i.e. surgically assisted rapid maxillary expansion (SARME). Various techniques for SARME have been developed. Most often, a Hyrax expander is cemented onto the maxillary first molars and premolars before the surgical treatment, which includes bilateral osteotomies performed from the piriform rims to the pterygomaxillary junction. A screw expansion of approximately 2 mm is performed directly after surgery, and the screw is then activated once or twice a day until the desired expansion has been achieved.

Treatment of scissors bite

The frequency of scissors bite including single teeth is 1 to 2%, and a scissors relationship is often related to single teeth; however, occasionally the complete lateral segment is involved. Scissors bite may occur unilaterally or bilaterally and can be associated with forced guidance of the mandible.

Treatment should start early to recreate occlusal contacts between premolars and molars, but also to avoid functional disturbances, such as lateral tooth interferences. If a single tooth is involved and without space deficiency for the displaced tooth, the use of inter-maxillary cross-elastics between the maxillary buccal and mandibular lingual tooth surfaces can be recommended.

In cases of a complete lateral segment in scissors bite or if a bilateral scissors bite is evident, a fixed appliance must be used to allow transversal contraction of the maxillary dentition and transversal expansion of the mandibular dentition as well as bite opening (Figure 5.23). The transversal contraction in the maxilla and expansion in the mandible can be supplemented with intermaxillary elastics.

Conclusions

Before treatment of inter jaw malocclusions, it is important to first perform a cephalometric analysis and, thereby provide a basis for an accurate differential diagnosis with respect to skeletal and dentoalveolar discrepancies.

Class II malocclusions, deep bite, posterior crossbite and scissors bite can be successfully treated either in the mixed or early permanent dentition.

To create successful treatment results, open bite and Class III malocclusions with skeletal origin are recommended to be treated in permanent dentition when growth has ceased. On the other hand, Class III malocclusion with dental origin (pseudo Class III malocclusion) can be treated in the mixed dentition. Open bite caused by sucking habits normally self-corrects if the habit terminates before 6 to 7 years of age.

REFERENCES

Andrésen, V., Häupl, K. and Petrik, L. (1957) *Funktionskieferorthopädie*. Johann Ambrosius Barth, Munich.

Ballanti, F., Lione, R., Baccetti, T. *et al.* (2010) Treatment and post treatment skeletal effects of rapid maxillary expansion investigated with low-dose computed tomography in growing subjects. Am J Orthod Dentofacial Orthop 138: 311–317.

Baratieri, C., Alves, M. Jr., de Souza, M.M. *et al.* (2011) Does rapid maxillary expansion have long-term effects on airway dimensions and breathing? Am J Orthod Dentofacial Orthop 140: 146–156.

Bass, N. (1982) Dentofacial orthopaedics in the correction of Class II malocclusion. Br J Orthod 9: 3–31.

Bazargani, F., Feldmann, I. and Bondemark, L. (2013) Three-dimensional analysis of effects of rapid maxillary expansion on facial sutures and bones. Angle Orthod 83: 1074–1082.

Bjerklin, K. (2000) Follow-up control of patients with unilateral posterior crossbite treated with expansion plates or the quad-helix appliance. J Orofac Orthop 61: 112–124.

Björk, A. (1955) Facial growth in man, studied with the aid of metallic implants. Acta Odont Scand 13: 9–34.

Bock, N.C., von Bremen, J. and Ruf, S. (2016) Stability of Class II fixed functional appliance therapy – a systematic review and meta-analysis. Eur J Orthod 38: 129–139.

Bondemark, L., Kurol, J. and Bernhold, M. (1994) Repelling magnets versus superelastic nickel titanium coils in simultaneous distal movement of maxillary first and second molars. Angle Orthod 64: 189–198.

Clark, W. (2010) Design and management of Twin Blocks: reflections after 30 years of clinical use. J Orthod 37: 209–216.

Cozzani, M., Guiducci, A., Mirenghi, S. et al. (2007) Arch width changes with a rapid maxillary expansion appliance anchored to the primary teeth. Angle Orthod 77: 296–302.

De Clerck, H. and Swennen, G.R. (2011) Success rate of miniplate anchorage for bone anchored maxillary protraction. Angle Orthod 81: 1010–1013.

Delaire, J. (1997) Maxillary development revisited: relevance to the orthopaedic treatment of class III malocclusions. Eur J Orthod 1997: 289–311.

de Oliveira, C.M. and Sheiham, A (2003) The relationship between normative orthodontic treatment need and oral health-related quality of life. Community Dent Oral Epidemiol 31: 426–436.

Dimberg, L., Lennartsson, B., Söderfeldt, B. et al. (2013) Malocclusions in children at 3 and 7 years of age: a longitudinal study. Eur J Orthod 35: 131–137.

Freeman, D.C., McNamara, J.A. Jr., Baccetti, T. et al. (2009) Long-term treatment effects of the FR-2 appliance of Fränkel. Am J Orthod Dentofacial Orthop 135: 570.e1–6.

Hart, T.R., Cousley, R.R., Fishman, L.S. et al. (2015) Dentoskeletal changes following mini-implant molar intrusion in anterior open bite patients. Angle Orthod 85: 941–948.

Heinig, N. and Göz, G. (2001) Clinical application and effects of the Forsus spring. A study of a new Herbst hybrid. J Orofac Orthop 62: 436–450.

Ludwig, B., Baumgaertel, S., Zorkun, B. et al. (2013) Application of a new viscoelastic finite element method model and analysis of miniscrew-supported hybrid hyrax treatment. Am J Orthod Dentofacial Orthop 143: 426–435.

Mandall, N., Di Biase, A., Littlewood, S. et al. (2010) Is early Class III protraction facemask treatment effective? A multicentre, randomized, controlled trial: 15-month follow-up. J Orthod 37: 149–161.

Ngan, P., Hu, A.M. and Fields, H.W. Jr. (1997) Treatment of Class III problems begins with differential diagnosis of anterior crossbites. Pediat Dent 19: 386–395.

Pancherz, H. and Ruf, S. (2008) The Herbst appliance – research-based clinical management. In: *The Herbst Appliance – research-based clinical management* (Eds H. Pancherz and S. Ruf), Berlin: Quintessence Publishing Co, Ltd.

Petrén, S., Bjerklin, K. and Bondemark, L. (2011) Stability of unilateral posterior crossbite correction in the mixed dentition: a randomized clinical trial with a 3-year follow-up. Am J Orthod Dentofacial Orthop 139: e73–81.

Petrén, S., Bjerklin, K., Marké, L.Å. et al. (2013) Early correction of posterior crossbite – a cost-minimization analysis. Eur J Orthod 35: 14–21.

Rabie, A.B. and Gu, Y. (1999) Management of preudo Class III malocclusion in southern Chinese children. Br Dent J 186: 183–187.

Teuscher, U. (1987) Class II treatment. Guidelines for class II treatment with the activator-headgear combination. Schweiz Monatsschr Zahnmed 97: 614–617.

Thilander, B. (1965) Chin-cup treatment for Angle Class III malocclusion. A longitudinal study. Trans Eur Orthod Soc 1965: 429–442.

Thilander, B. and Myrberg, N. (1973) The prevalence of malocclusion in Swedish schoolchildren. Scand J Dent Res 81: 12–21.

Thilander, B., Wahlund, S. and Lennartsson, B. (1984) The effect of early interceptive treatment in children with posterior cross-bite. Eur J Orthod 6: 25–34.

Thilander, B. and Lennartsson, B. (2002) A study of children with unilateral posterior crossbite, treated and untreated, in the deciduous dentition – occlusal and skeletal characteristics of significance in predicting the long-term outcome. J Orofac Orthop 65: 371–383.

Thilander, B., Persson, M. and Adolfsson U. (2005) Roentgen-cephalometric standards for a Swedish population. A longitudinal study between the ages of 5 and 31 years. Eur J Orthod 27: 370–389.

Thiruvenkatachari, B., Harrison, J.E., Worthington, H.V. et al. (2013) Early orthodontic treatment for children with prominent upper front teeth reduces more the incidence of trauma than providing one course of treatment when the child is in early adolescence. Cochrane Database Syst Rev 11: Art. No.: CD003452. doi: 10.1002/14651858.CD003452.pub3.

van Beek, H. (1982) Overjet correction by a combined headgear and activator. Eur J Orthod 4: 279–290.

Vargervik, K. and Harvold, E.P. (1985) Response to activator treatment in Class II malocclusions. Am J Orthod 88: 242–251.

Weissheimer, A., de Menezes, L.M., Mezomo, M. et al. (2011) Immediate effects of rapid maxillary expansion with Haas-type and Hyrax-type expanders: a randomized clinical trial. Am J Orthod Dentofacial Orthop 140: 366–376.

Wiedel, A.P. (2015) Fixed or removable appliance for early orthodontic treatment of functional anterior crossbite. Swed Dent J, Suppl 238: 10–72. (Thesis)

Zymperdikas, V.F., Koretsi, V., Papageorgiou, S.N. et al. (2016) Treatment effects of fixed functional appliances in patients with Class II malocclusion: a systematic review and meta-analysis. Eur J Orthod 38: 113–126.

CHAPTER 6
Crowding of teeth

Krister Bjerklin and Lars Bondemark

Key topics

- Model analysis
- Treatment strategies
- Expansion of dental arches to gain space
- Reduction of tooth material by extraction or enamel reduction of teeth

Learning objectives

- To be able, in a model analysis, to evaluate the arch length, arch width and form, amount of crowding and size of the apical base
- To understand treatment strategies for crowding of teeth in the primary, mixed and permanent dentition
- To know when and how to expand the dental arches to solve crowding of teeth
- To know when and how to solve crowding with extractions
- To know when and how to assess enamel reduction to solve crowding of teeth

Essential Orthodontics, First Edition. Birgit Thilander, Krister Bjerklin and Lars Bondemark.
© 2018 John Wiley & Sons Ltd. Published 2018 by John Wiley & Sons Ltd.

Introduction

Crowding of teeth is one of the most common malocclusions with a frequency of about 25%. Crowding of teeth in the jaw is often generalised but can be local in the anterior or posterior region of the jaw, and then with the latest erupted teeth; for instance, the maxillary canine will be buccally displaced or a second premolar will be dislocated lingually in the dental arch. Moreover, premature loss of deciduous molars and the resulting mesial migration of permanent molars will develop crowding in the premolar and canine region.

Crowding of teeth is more frequent in the mandible than in the maxilla, and crowding in the mandible is often combined with deep bite. The need for treatment is often owed to aesthetic reasons, and evidence exists that untreated crowded anterior teeth will result in negative effects on oral-health-related quality of life.

Minor crowding of teeth is considered a normal condition; particularly, in the mandibular incisor region, minor crowding is found in almost all individuals and this crowding increases with age.

In treatment planning for crowding of teeth, there are several factors to consider:

■ the severity of crowding;
■ the form of the alveolar arches, including the apical bases;
■ whether it is possible to expand the dental arch to gain space or whether reduction of tooth material should be performed;
■ the skeletal relationships of the face;
■ the remaining facial growth;
■ the shape of the lips and the lip-seal;
■ hereditary factors (small dental arches versus large-sized teeth).

Model analysis

To more precisely evaluate the extent of crowding, arch form and the apical bases of the jaws, it is recommended to take study casts of the jaws and make a model analysis. On the study casts, it is easy with the aid of a sliding calliper to measure arch length, arch width, amount of crowding of teeth, overjet and overbite and rotation

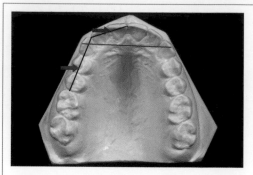

Figure 6.1 Arch length, from the mesial surface of the first permanent molar to the distal surface of the lateral incisor (the line at the blue arrow). The anterior length represents the distance between the mesial surface of the canine and the midline of the dental arch (the line at the red arrow). The intercanine width is the distance between the crown tips of the canines (the red line).

of teeth (Figure 6.1). The model analysis also includes determination of the size of the apical base; dental arch form; the sagittal, vertical and transversal relation between the jaws; and the relation between the midlines in the maxilla and the mandible.

Over all, the crowding of teeth is closely related to the size of the teeth and the adequacy of bony support for the teeth in the jaws. The volume of the alveolar bone that is on a level with the root apices of the teeth is called the apical base. When the alveolar process of the jaw is undersized, and thereby does not have enough space for the roots of the teeth, the disproportion is called a small apical base, which often results in proclined incisors and crowding of the anterior teeth (Figure 6.2a). The opposite is a large apical base (Figure 6.2b), which means that the alveolar process of the jaw is oversized, resulting in vertical positions of the teeth and spacing (Lundström, 1923).

Crowding of teeth in the anterior part of the jaws can be evaluated by using Little's irregularity index, whereby the distances between the contact points on adjacent teeth from canine to canine are measured (Little, 1975).

It must be emphasised, however, that in addition to the extent of crowding of teeth, arch form and the apical base, the face in profile,

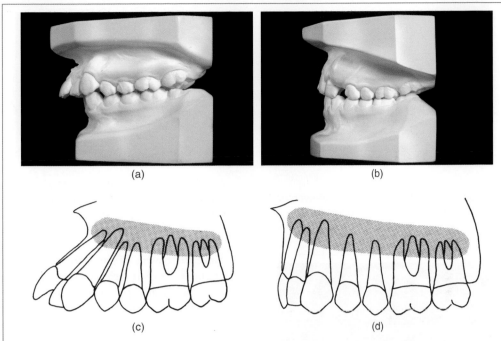

Figure 6.2 Models with a small apical base, shaded area in the drawing (a,c), the skeletal base is not sufficiently large for the teeth and therefore the incisors are proclined. A large apical base (b,d) resulting in vertical positions of the teeth.

skeletal relationships of the face, the shape of the lips and lip seal, as well as remaining growth, must also be considered in treatment planning of crowding.

Orthodontic appliances

In the permanent dentition, both extraction and non-extraction treatments, require treatment with fixed appliances, multibracket techniques, with the brackets on the labial surfaces or on the lingual surfaces to achieve derotated teeth, parallel roots, Class I occlusion and a stable occlusion.

A great number of fixed appliance systems are on the market, as well as several different anchorage systems. Temporary anchorage devices (TADs), such as mini screws and fixed anchorage plates, were developed at the end of the 20th century. Furthermore, intermaxillary elastics such as Class II or Class III elastics may be necessary to attain stable occlusion and a good aesthetic result. The use of different

appliances is described in detail in other textbooks, for example, multibracket techniques by Bennett and McLaughlin (2014).

Sometimes removable appliances such as the Invisalign technique can be used. This technique uses a series of very thin aligners. The practically invisible aligners are individually manufactured and are changed every 2 to 3 weeks to the next set of aligners. The Invisalign treatment is performed during 1 to 2 years, and is mainly recommended for adults or non-growing patients.

Treatment strategies

Primary dentition – mixed dentition

Treatment of crowding in deciduous dentition is seldom indicated. In mixed dentition, slight anterior crowding (2–3 mm) (Figure 6.3) at the time of eruption of the incisors can be followed without treatment, since self-correction of the crowding occurs. The normal growth of the

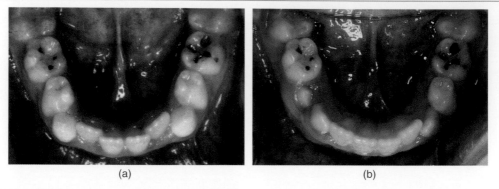

(a)   (b)

Figure 6.3 Slight anterior mandibular incisor crowding in the mixed dentition (a) and the crowding will most often self-correct during the development to the permanent dentition as observed in this case (b).

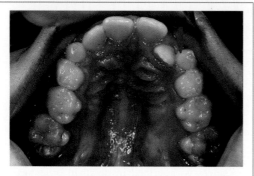

Figure 6.4 A moderate anterior crowding, and in this case it is recommended to slice off the mesial surfaces of the deciduous left canine (blue arrow) to create extra space for the lateral incisor to self-align.

jaws and increased arch length due to proclined eruption direction of the permanent incisors as well as increased intercanine distance contributes to the self-correction of crowding.

When moderate anterior crowding (3–4 mm) exists (Figure 6.4) and if the lateral incisors have erupted in a rotated and palatal direction with an obvious risk of ending up in an anterior crossbite, the mesial surface of the deciduous canine can be sliced off to create extra space for alignment of the lateral incisors. The crowding is now transferred distally and it is then later appropriate to slice the deciduous second molar mesially in order to guide the erupting premolars into their correct positions.

Since the crowns of the second deciduous molars are wider than the succeeding premolars (Leeway space), this space may also contribute to correct the crowding. In the mandible, the Leeway space is 2 to 3 mm and 1 to 2 mm in the maxilla.

Prediction of space for premolars and permanent canines in the mixed dentition can be carried out. All prediction methods have shown to have errors. Generally, in children who have mesio-distal widths of the maxillary incisors within normal range and normal positions, the distance from the mesial surface of the first permanent molar to the distal surface of the permanent lateral incisor is estimated at 22 mm in the maxilla and 21 mm in the mandible. These assumptions of 22 and 21 mm are based on the premolars, on average, having a mesio-distal width of 7 mm, the maxillary canine 8 mm and the mandibular canine 7 mm.

When crowding is severe, more than 8 mm in the jaw (Figure 6.5), there is an indication to remove the primary canines in order to make it possible for the incisors to erupt or to reduce crowding of erupted incisors. In most of these cases, a serial or guided extraction therapy ending up with extraction of premolars is appropriate, especially if Class I malocclusions with normal overbite and a Class I skeletal relation are also evident. Kjellgren (1948) published an article about serial extraction as a corrective procedure in dental orthopaedic therapy. Later, many studies have been published on this topic (Dale and Dale, 2012). In the serial

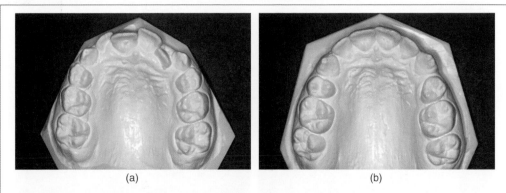

Figure 6.5 The maxillary arch of a 10-year-old girl showing crowded incisors (a). Some years later (b), after extraction of the primary canines and extraction of the first premolars. The incisors are spontaneously corrected and only a short period with fixed appliance remains to correct the left premolar and to close the small spacings.

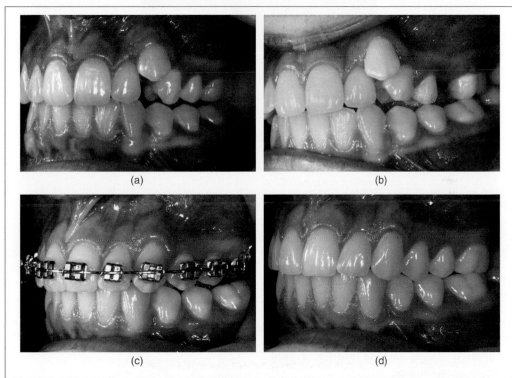

Figure 6.6 The maxillary premolars and molars on the left side have moved mesially, resulting in a Class II malocclusion and a crowded maxillary left canine (a). After distal molar movement of 4 mm during 6 months (b) and a subsequent multibracket fixed appliance (c). The result one year after treatment (d).

extraction approach, it is important to remove the mandibular first premolars before the permanent canines have erupted to avoid further crowding of the incisors. This also means that the mandibular first primary molars should be extracted to accelerate the eruption of the first premolars. It must be noted that a final period of fixed appliance therapy is needed in some of the cases to secure a fully satisfactory alignment and occlusion.

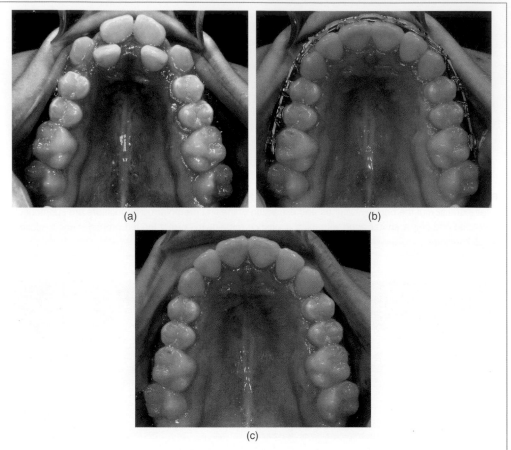

(a)

(b)

(c)

Figure 6.7 In this crowded case (a), transversal expansion with a multibracket fixed appliance has been achieved (b), and a final good alignment of the teeth has been created (c).

Permanent dentition

In principle, crowding can be solved by either expanding the dental arches to gain space or by reducing the tooth material. Regardless of whether expansion of dental arches or reduction of tooth material shall be performed, the most common treatment method involves a fixed multibracket technique.

Expansion of the dental arch to gain space

Normally, expansion of the dental arch can be created by sagittal expansion, i.e. proclination of incisors and/or distal movement of posterior teeth (Figure 6.6). Transversal expansion is also possible to assess increasing space in the jaws

(Figure 6.7). To succeed with expansion treatment, the total crowding of teeth should not amount to more than 6 to 7 mm in the jaw, and the apical base should be normal and absolutely not small. Most often, a fixed appliance is inserted in both jaws for expansion, but removable appliances using the Invisalign technique are also used (Figure 6.8).

Distal molar movement is the treatment of choice in the maxilla for sagittal expansion, especially when mesial migration of the molars has occurred. The distal molar movement can be performed with either an extra oral appliance, i.e. headgear or with intra oral appliances of different types. It has been shown that the intra oral appliances are more effective than the extra oral appliances to move the molars

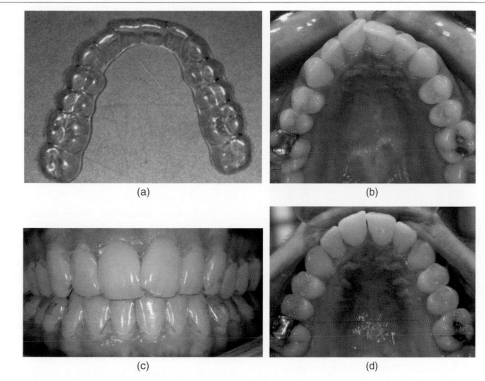

(a)

(b)

(c)

(d)

Figure 6.8 In the Invisalign technique, a series of aligners are used, and in (a) one of the aligners. Before treatment and a slight crowding of maxillary central incisors (b). The aligners inserted in both jaws (c), and after 4 months of treatment, the central incisors are almost fully aligned (d). Photos with permission of Dr Thor Henrikson.

distally (Bondemark and Karlsson, 2005). Two to three millimetres of distal molar movement is realistic; furthermore, 1 to 2 mm can be gained by derotation of the first molars.

Various non-compliance intra oral fixed appliances for distal molar movement have been introduced, and the most recent appliances use TADs as anchorage systems combined with fixed appliances (Figure 6.9). There are also distal movement systems consisting of a force-generating unit including superelastic coils, an anchorage unit usually comprising premolars or deciduous molars, and an anchorage Nance button.

In the mandible with limited crowding and deep bite, multibracket fixed appliances can be used for reduction of the curve of Spee, together with bite opening by incisor proclination. However, proclination of the mandibular

incisors must be performed with caution, since too much incisor proclination is associated with a strong tendency of relapse.

Reduction of tooth material

Reduction of tooth material involves extractions of teeth or reduction of the mesio-distal width of the teeth by enamel reduction.

Extraction of teeth When extractions of teeth are performed to solve crowding, the extractions are always followed by treatment with a multibracket fixed appliance in both jaws, while removable appliances – for example, the Invisalign technique – are seldom appropriate as a treatment option. In principle, the teeth are aligned and moved within the alveolar process into good occlusion and contact relationships

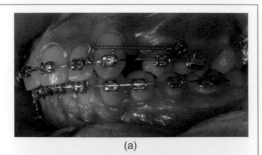

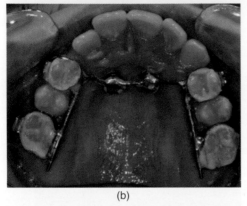

(a)

(b)

Figure 6.9 In (a), a miniscrew (TAD) has been inserted between the roots of the maxillary second premolar and first molar to create reinforced anchorage during space closure. In (b), two TADs (miniscrews) have been inserted in the palate for anchorage support during distal molar movement.

For instance, teeth severely damaged due to caries, fillings, trauma, hypomineralization or root resorption caused by impacted canines must be taken into consideration. In such cases, teeth other than the first premolars can be selected for extraction.

Extraction of lateral incisors is appropriate when an erupting canine has generated root resorption of the lateral incisor or when the lateral incisors are small or peg shaped.

Extraction of canines is rare, but may be necessary if the canine is positioned or impacted far out of its correct position.

If the first molars are badly damaged, or show severe molar incisor hypomineralization (MIH), it is more appropriate to extract such teeth. Moreover, in cases of crowding in combination with open bite, it may be preferable to extract first or second molars.

One or more mandibular incisors are recommended to be extracted on special recommendation, i.e. severe crowding of the mandibular incisors or when marked gingival recessions are evident, especially if the incisor is proclined.

Enamel reduction When crowding is slight, or if tooth discrepancies are evident, it is often advisable to reduce the mesio-distal width of the crowded teeth. The amount of enamel reduction depends on the crown morphology. Normally, 0.1 to 0.2 mm on each surface can be reduced; thus, if enamel reduction is assessed for 6 teeth (4 incisors and 2 canines), this will result in a 1.2 to 2.4 mm gain of space. Enamel reduction can also be combined with sagittal and/or transversal expansion. The crowding is eliminated by expansion and enamel reduction, and simultaneously the contact points between the teeth will be broader, promoting more stable inter-tooth contacts.

The enamel reduction can be performed directly by an air-rotor stripping diamond disk or a metal-diamond strip followed by a polishing disc or strip and a polishing paste (Figure 6.11). To increase the control of the enamel reduction, interproximal separation of the teeth can be recommended before the enamel reduction procedure is performed.

(Figure 6.10). It is also important to secure that the extraction spaces are devoted to eliminate the crowding and aligning the teeth after removal of the teeth. Thus, unwanted tooth movements and anchorage loss must be prevented. The anchorage planning involves how to distribute the forces to the different teeth involved and to promote the best space closure possible. Of course, there is considerable variation in the anchorage requirement for individual cases.

In most cases, the extraction of first premolars is selected for removal, since these teeth often are close to the crowded teeth, and first premolar extractions result in the most effective treatment. However, it may sometimes be advantageous to extract other teeth.

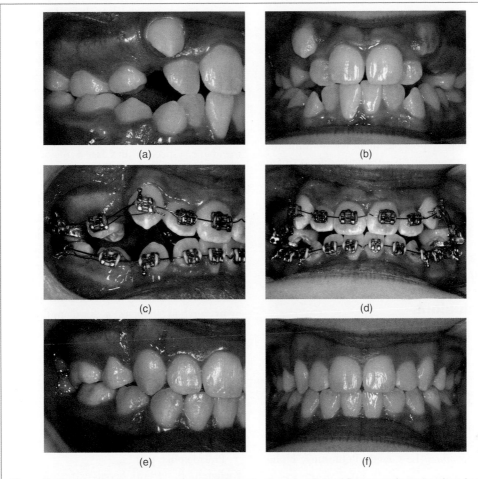

Figure 6.10 In (a, b), shows a severe crowded case solved by bilateral first premolar extractions in each jaw followed by bimaxillary fixed multibracket appliance (c, d). The final result (e, f).

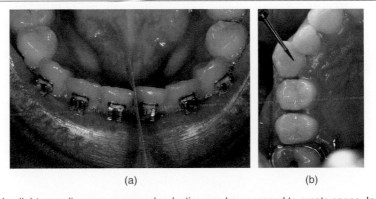

Figure 6.11 In slight crowding cases, enamel reduction can be assessed to create space. In (a), the reduction is performed by a diamond strip and in (b), by an air-rotor drill.

Adult patients

Treatment of adults with crowding of teeth varies more than with treatment of children. Some patients only want to have corrections in the aesthetic area, while others want full fixed orthodontic treatment. Moreover, in adults, a careful examination must be done, even if some patients do not want to have a comprehensive orthodontic treatment. It is important to know what is possible in order to fulfil the patient's requirements. Aesthetic improvement is the main reason for adult patients with crowding, but occlusal stability and chewing comfort are also reasons why adult patients seek orthodontic treatment. More adults than children and adolescents want to have 'invisible' orthodontic appliances, such as lingual appliances or Invisalign treatment.

Conclusions

For evaluation of the amount of crowding, arch form and the apical bases of the jaws, it is recommended to take study casts of the jaws and make a model analysis. In addition to the extent of crowding of teeth, arch form and the apical base, the face in profile, skeletal relationships of the face, the shape of the lips and lip seal, as well as remaining growth, must be considered for treatment planning of crowding.

In mixed dentition when the crowding is severe, a serial extraction procedure is recommendable, especially if Class I malocclusions with normal overbite and a Class I skeletal relation are also evident.

In permanent dentition, the crowding can be solved by either expanding the dental arches to gain space or by reducing the tooth material by tooth extraction or by interproximal enamel reduction. Regardless of whether expansion of the dental arches or reduction of tooth material is performed, the most common treatment method involves a fixed multibracket technique.

REFERENCES

Bennett, J.C. and McLaughlin, R.P. (2014) *Fundamentals of Orthodontic Treatment Mechanics*. Le Grande Publishing, Hong Kong.

Bondemark, L. and Karlsson, I. (2005) Extra oral vs intra oral appliance for distal movement of maxillary first molars: a randomized controlled trial. Angle Orthod 75: 699–706.

Dale, J.G. and Dale, H.C. (2012) Interceptive guidance of occlusion, with emphasis on diagnosis. In *Orthodontics: Current Principles and Techniques*, 5th edition (Eds T.M. Graber, R.L. Vanarsdall and K.W.L. Vig), 5, Elsevier Mosby, Philadelphia, p. 423.

Kjellgren, B. (1948) Serial extraction as a corrective procedure in dental orthopedic therapy. Acta Odontol Scand 8(1): 17–43.

Little, R.M. (1975) The irregularity index. A quantitative score of mandibular anterior alignment. Am J Orthod 68: 554–563.

Lundström, A. (1923) Malocclusions of the teeth regarded as a problem in connection with the apical base. Int J Orthod 11.

CHAPTER 7
Spacing of teeth

Birgit Thilander and Krister Bjerklin

Key topics

- Median diastema
- Missing maxillary incisors
- Pathological migration of teeth
- Congenitally missing premolars
- Partial edentulous dentitions
- General spacing of teeth

Learning objectives

- To be able to discuss treatment principles in patients with a median diastema
- To be able to describe treatment alternatives in patients with missing maxillary incisors
- To understand problems, associated with orthodontic treatment in patients, treated for periodontitis
- To understand the importance of multidisciplinary co-operation in treatment of patients with partial edentulous dentition

Essential Orthodontics, First Edition. Birgit Thilander, Krister Bjerklin and Lars Bondemark.
© 2018 John Wiley & Sons Ltd. Published 2018 by John Wiley & Sons Ltd.

Introduction

Excess of space in the dental arch is diagnosed as a generalised spacing or a local divergence, often observed in the maxillary anterior region, as a median diastema, traumatic loss of central incisors, or congenital absence of lateral incisors. Furthermore, spacing is observed in aging individuals, due to pathological migration of teeth caused by periodontitis. Finally, adult individuals with partial edentulous jaws demand pre-prosthetic orthodontic treatment from functional aspects. Thus, indication for orthodontic treatment in subjects with spacing of teeth exists for aesthetic reasons, but also for facilitating prosthetic restorations with optimal occlusal stability.

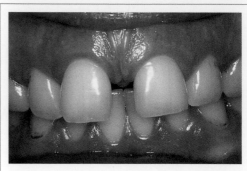

Figure 7.1 Median diastema with a hypertrophic frenulum.

Median diastema

A maxillary diastema is common in early mixed dentition and can be regarded as a normal feature in connection with eruption of the central incisors. In most cases, there is a progressive reduction, especially at the eruption of the lateral incisors and the canines. In permanent dentition, the frequency is about 4% in a Swedish population (Thilander and Myrberg, 1973).

A hypertrophic labial frenulum (thick and/or attached to the gingival margin) has been debated as a causative factor or a consequence of a persistent diastema (Figure 7.1). It is not in itself a hindrance to spontaneous closure of the diastema, but excision hastens the spontaneous closure, especially in the 'divergent type'. The frenotomy should be performed before the eruption of the lateral incisors in order to create enough space for them in the dental arch. However, in cases with 'parallel' central incisors or generalised spacing, as well as in adolescents, spontaneous closure should not be expected (Figure 7.1). Such cases need appliance therapy.

Before orthodontic closure of the diastema, it is important to verify by radiographs that no obstacles (e.g. mesiodens, odontoma) exist between the central incisors, and if occurring, they should be removed. Maxillary median diastemas are relatively simple to close with fixed appliances, which at the same time ensure adequate root paralleling and correct torque of the

incisors. Tipping of the teeth with removable appliances should normally be avoided, since the roots may be left diverging, which commonly results in space reopening.

Adult patients frequently demand a closure of the anterior diastema for aesthetic reasons. The treatment principles in general are the same as for adolescents. However, in adults, compromise solutions can be chosen. Median diastema closure is relatively simple if the overjet will allow a palatally shift of the incisors (Figure 7.2). If an overjet reduction is impossible, the teeth must be moved into ideally separated positions and the crowns built up with porcelain veneers or composite resins. Diastema closure needs bodily movements to avoid tipping, while fixed appliances must be used to control both crown and root positions. Due to the risk of relapse, retention appliances must be used for a long time, and in some cases even require permanent retention.

Missing maxillary incisors

Missing teeth, because of trauma or congenital absence, generally affect the maxillary anterior region. Aesthetic improvement is the real desire of the patient. Treatment solutions include orthodontic space closure, auto-transplantation or prosthetic replacement (bonded or fixed dental bridges, or implant-supported crowns). All alternatives have their advantages as well as disadvantages and proper decisions should be made already in young ages. A comprehensive treatment plan often implies a compromise in the

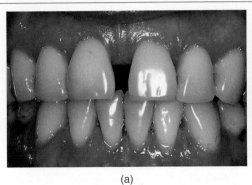 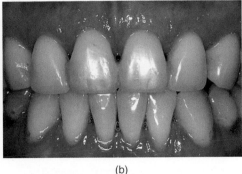

(a)   (b)

Figure 7.2 A median diastema before treatment (a) and the result after closure with a fixed orthodontic appliance (b).

individual case, and should be discussed in a multidisciplinary team. Then, the patient and his/her parents should be thoroughly informed of each step of the total treatment procedure.

Central incisors

Missing maxillary central incisors are usually caused by a traumatic injury. The immediate measure, following the trauma, is descried in some textbooks (Andreasen, 1992), while this present chapter focuses on the orthodontic problem.

Space closure by moving a tooth through the mid-palatal suture has shown to be unsuccessful in an experimental study in beagle dogs (Follin *et al.*, 1984). Hence, the gap should be closed from both sides, resulting in three incisors. It is, however, important to correct the axial inclination and mesio-distal position when a lateral incisor is used to replace a central one. Some patients may accept such an alternative, if the incisors are of the same size and their axial inclination has been corrected.

Autotransplantation of a premolar to this area in young patients with an optimal stage of three-quarters root development (Slagsvold and Bjercke, 1978) has shown good long-term results (Czochrowska *et al.*, 2002; Kvint *et al.*, 2010) (Figure 7.3). Replacement by a single tooth implant-supported crown is usually the alternative in young adults, thus leaving the adjacent teeth intact. However, in some cases, a fixed dental prosthesis is another alternative in adult patients. Resin-retained construction,

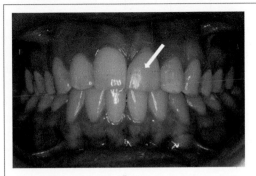

Figure 7.3 A maxillary left central incisor was replaced by a transplanted premolar 13 years ago because of trauma. The white arrow points at the restored premolar.

serving as a space maintainer during the dental development while awaiting the final treatment decision, is the best alternative in young and adolescent individuals.

Lateral incisors

The frequency of congenitally missing maxillary lateral incisors is 1 to 2% and the treatment alternatives are the same as for central incisors. Autotransplantation of a premolar to this region may be an alternative in the young patient. However, the width of the crown of the premolar is 1 to 2 mm larger than that of a lateral incisor, and thus is not the optimal alternative. Instead, the orthodontic closure or orthodontic opening of the space for prosthetic replacement, are the two treatment alternatives.

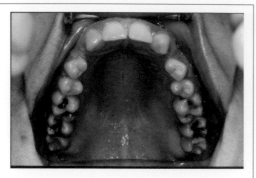

Figure 7.4 Agenesis of the lateral incisors. The maxillary canines have erupted close to and in contact with the central incisors.

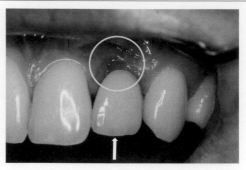

Figure 7.5 The implant-supported crown in infraocclusion (white arrow) 5 years after the implant has been inserted in an 18-year-old boy. Also, note the reduction of the marginal gingiva (yellow ring).

The decision should be made in the early mixed dentition. In some individuals, when the canine has a mesial eruption direction, it is possible to guide the canine into a position in contact with the central incisor (Figure 7.4)

Orthodontic space closure aims to allow a canine to replace the missing lateral incisor, and is the best alternative from the periodontal point of view. However, opponents point to dental aesthetics, as the canine is broader than the lateral, even in the palatal-buccal direction and hence may become prominent, its anatomy requires reshaping, and it has a darker yellow colour than the incisors. Such colour discrepancy was found to be the major cause of dissatisfaction among individuals who had received orthodontic closure (Robertsson and Mohlin, 2000). Composite reshaping and bleaching are alternatives to compensate for those problems. Thus, many factors have to be considered in space closure and in adult patients, compromises have to be chosen.

Replacement by an implant-supported crown is often recommended as the best treatment option due to its high capacity for osseointegration and moreover leaves the adjacent teeth untouched (Figure 5.5). The orthodontic treatment is to gain sufficient space for the implant, even in the apical area, which may be problematic because of the dimension of the implant. Overexpansion has been recommended, but this will involve tipping of the teeth, resulting in a reduced space of the apical area.

It is well-known that dental implants should not be inserted until the permanent dentition is fully erupted and the craniofacial growth is completed, to avoid infraocclusion of the implant-supported crown (Thilander *et al.*, 1994). However, complete growth (registered by body height and cephalometric registrations) and complete dental development will not guarantee avoidance of infra-occlusion, as shown in a 10-year follow-up study (Thilander *et al.*, 2001). The mean increase of the vertical dimension was 0.98 mm during the whole observation period (with individual variations from 0.1–2.2 mm) and understood as a continuous eruption of the adjacent teeth. These findings agree with longitudinal studies on dentoalveolar development (Iseri and Solow, 1996; Thilander, 2009). During the last few years, infra-positioned implant-supported crowns have been reported, even with implant placement in older adults, and it has been speculated about a relationship with a type of craniofacial morphology. However, in another long-term study of implants (Andersson *et al.*, 2013), small degrees of infraposition were observed, but no clear relationship between degree of infraposition and facial shape was possible to establish. Hence, we must remember that slow physiological changes of the occlusion take place over years.

It is important to also have an understanding of some periodontal complications round the implant. Frequent lack of gingival papillary

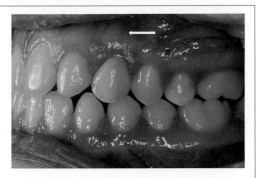

Figure 7.6 The maxillary left canine has replaced the missed lateral incisor and adjacent to the canine is an implant-supported crown (canine) with a discoloured mucosa along the implant (white arrow) two years after treatment.

filling might cause an unaesthetic appearance. As reported in the 10-year follow-up study (Thilander *et al.*, 2001), an apical shift of the soft tissue margin with a discoloured mucosa was observed (Figure 7.6). This indicates loss of marginal bone support on the labial aspect of the implant and is further verified by mucosal retraction. A reduction of the marginal bone level at the adjacent teeth was also noted. The shorter the distance between the implant and the adjacent tooth surfaces, the larger was the reduction of the marginal bone level. Thus, even if a dental implant in the maxillary incisor area is recommended as the best treatment option due to its high capacity for osseo-integration, it is difficult to decide whether it is the best alternative in the individual case, due to the aesthetic and periodontal outcome.

Removable appliances to replace one or both laterals are often rejected by the patient. Full-coverage fixed dental prosthesis requires grinding of tooth substance, with a high risk of pulp damage in young adult patients. In these cases, a resin-retained fixed dental prosthesis may be an alternative. The success of these restorations is directly related to the efficiency of the bonding ability, and reported survivals vary widely (Van Dalen *et al.*, 2004). However, regardless of which prosthodontic procedure is chosen, pre-prosthetic orthodontic treatment is usually necessary to gain sufficient space for the lateral incisors and to upright the adjacent teeth.

Pathological migration of teeth due to periodontitis

Pathological tooth migration can involve a single tooth or a group of teeth and result in a median diastema or general spacing, often combined with infrabony pockets and/or proclination of the maxillary incisors. The overall treatment for those patients often involves orthodontic realignment of the teeth to re-establish satisfactory occlusion and aesthetic conditions. After treatment of the periodontal disease, including elimination of plaque, retention factors and deep gingival pockets, the orthodontic treatment can start.

Clinical and radiographic observations from animal experimental studies have shown that orthodontic treatment in patients, treated for periodontitis, can be successfully performed, provided the following programme is followed:

■ the orthodontic appliance must be properly designed to permit proper plaque control;
■ proper anchorage of the teeth must be selected regarding the degree of their bony support;
■ light forces should be used as the alveolar bone support is reduced;
■ thorough clinical and radiographic assessments should be made to check that adverse effect does not occur;
■ the occlusion should be adjusted to avoid interferences;
■ the oral hygiene, including pocket probing, shall be checked at each dental visit.

Spacing in the posterior areas of the dentition

In patients with partial edentulous dentitions, because of congenitally absence or extraction of teeth, orthodontic treatment should often be performed, especially due to functional aspects.

Congenitally missing premolars

The frequency of congenitally missing premolars is 2 to 3%, with the highest frequency for mandibular second premolars. It is important to remember that the diagnosis agenesis can be verified firstly at the age of 9 to 10 years.

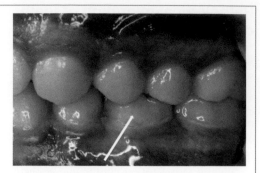

Figure 7.7 A transplanted maxillary third molar (white arrow) that has replaced the missed mandibular second premolar.

Orthodontic space closure by guiding the erupting teeth into a stable occlusion is a good choice in children, especially in the maxilla with its high space closing potential. This alternative, however, is more complex in adolescents and young adults because of an interlocking occlusion that often needs compensatory treatment in the opposite dental arch.

In severe crowding cases, the primary mandibular second molar can be extracted and the available space used to relieve crowding or retract anterior teeth, or both. If the extraction can be made early, at 11 years of age or earlier, before eruption of the second permanent molar, good spontaneous improvement and space closure often occurs.

To avoid tipping of the teeth, bodily orthodontic movements must be used with light forces to avoid interdental folds with sub-lethal damage to the gingiva. Space closure is time-consuming and the alternative dental implant treatment should be considered.

Autotransplantation of a maxillary third molar is an option in replacing a missing mandibular second premolar. The width of a maxillary third molar is most often equal to a mandibular second primary molar (Figure 7.7). The best time for transplantation is when the third molar has a root development of three-quarters of its length.

Implant-supporting crowns can be a good choice in replacing missing premolars in young adults and adult patients, as shown in a 10-year follow-up study (Thilander *et al.*, 2001). All implant-supported crowns in this area were in good occlusion, despite a step (varying between 0.2 and 2.1 mm) to the adjacent molar because of a continuous eruption of the adjacent molar, according to the findings by Sarnäs and Solow (1980) and Iseri and Solow (1996). An implant, replacing a missing mandibular premolar, needs sufficient bone volume, not only in the mesio-distal, but above all in the bucco-lingual direction. Early extraction of a primary molar, associated with congenital absence of a permanent successor, will cause an hour-glass-shaped alveolar bone, which may jeopardize implant placement, if not bone augmentation is performed.

Partial edentulous dentitions

Tipped molars and reduced alveolar height are frequently found in adults after performed extractions in earlier ages. By positioning the teeth towards or into the edentulous area, improved aesthetic and functional results can be obtained with optimal occlusal stability and chewing comfort. A comprehensive analysis and treatment plan should be based on a discussion between the orthodontist and the dentist who is responsible for the prosthetic procedure. The prosthodontic opinion has to be evaluated against orthodontic aspects, for example the individual anatomy of the tissue area in which the tooth (teeth) is moved into. An optimal treatment goal for the patient should be made, also considering finances. A schedule including the various steps of the treatment is presented to the patient, who will be informed in detail about the time of each step of the total procedure.

General spacing of teeth

General spacing is a distributed spreading of the teeth with diastemas from premolar to premolar in an otherwise normal occlusion. Small tooth size together with a large apical base is the cause to the anomaly. Closure of the gaps or realignment of teeth for prosthetic replacement is the treatment alternatives. Both need fixed appliances in both jaws during a long treatment period with a great risk for relapse. Consequently, a prolonged or permanent retention is necessary.

REFERENCES

Andersson, B., Bergenblock, S., Fürst, B. *et al.* (2013) Long-term function of single-implant restorations: A 17- to 19-year follow-up study on implant infra-position related to the shape of the face and patient's satisfaction. Clin Implant Dent Relat Res 15: 471–480.

Andreasen, J. (1992) *Atlas of Replantation and Autotransplantation of Teeth.* Medioglobe, Switzerland.

Czochrowska, E., Stenvik, A., Bjercke, B. *et al.* (2002) Outcome of tooth transplantation: survival and success rates 17–41 years post-treatment. Am J Orthod Dentofacial Orthop 121: 110–119.

Follin, M., Ericsson, I. and Thilander, B. (1984) Orthodontic tooth movement of maxillary incisors through midpalatal suture area: an experimental study in dogs. Eur J Orthod 6: 237–246.

Iseri, H. and Solow, B. (1996) Continued eruption of maxillary incisors and first molars in girls from 9 to 25 years, studied by the implant method. Eur J Orthod 18: 245–256.

Kvint, S., Lindsten, R., Magnusson, A. *et al.* (2010) Autotransplantation of teeth in 215 patients. A follow-up study. Angle Orthod 80: 446–451.

Robertsson, S. and Mohlin, B. (2000) The congenitally missing upper incisor. A retrospective study of orthodontic space closure versus restorative treatment. Eur J Orthod 22: 697–710.

Sarnäs, K-V. and Solow, B. (1980) Early adult changes in the skeletal and soft-tissue profile. Eur J Orthod 2: 1–12.

Slagsvold, O. and Bjercke, B. (1978) Applicability of autotransplantation in cases of missing upper anterior teeth. Am J Orthod 74: 410–421.

Thilander, B. and Myrberg, N. (1973) The prevalence of malocclusion in Swedish schoolchildren. Scand J Dent Res 81: 12–21.

Thilander, B., Ödman, J., Gröndahl, K. *et al.* (1994) Osseointegrated implants in adolescents. An alternative in replacing missing teeth? Eur J Orthod 16: 84–95.

Thilander, B., Ödman, J. and Lekholm, U. (2001) Orthodontic aspects of the use of oral implants in adolescents: a 10-year follow-up study. Eur J Orthod 23: 715–731.

Thilander, B. (2009) Dentoalveolar development in subjects with normal occlusion. A longitudinal study between the ages of 5 and 31 years. Eur J Orthod 31: 109–120.

Van Dalen, A., Feilzer, A. and Kleveraan, C. (2004) A literature review of two-unit cantilevered FPDs. Int J Prosthodont 17: 281–284.

CHAPTER 8
Malposition of single teeth

Krister Bjerklin

Key topics

- Infraocclusion of primary molars
- Ectopic eruption of maxillary first permanent molars
- Impacted maxillary canines
- Supernumerary anterior teeth – mesiodens

Learning objectives

- To know how to manage infraocclusion of primary molars
- To know how to manage ectopic eruption of maxillary first permanent molars
- To be able to diagnose and managing impacted maxillary canines at the appropriate time
- To know risks with impacted maxillary canines regarding root resorptions of adjacent teeth

Essential Orthodontics, First Edition. Birgit Thilander, Krister Bjerklin and Lars Bondemark.
© 2018 John Wiley & Sons Ltd. Published 2018 by John Wiley & Sons Ltd.

Introduction

Developmental disturbances of teeth are anomalies of position or eruption path. Form, shape and number of teeth are other tooth disturbances. It has been suggested that such developmental anomalies are all micro symptoms of an inheritable developmental disturbance due to a general disturbance of the developmental tooth structures (Pfeiffer, 1974; Hoffmeister, 1977).

Eruption disturbance, such as impacted maxillary canines, is associated with ectopic eruption of maxillary first permanent molars, infraocclusion of primary molars, peg-shaped or congenitally missing maxillary lateral incisors and agenesis of mandibular second premolars (Bjerklin et al., 1992; Baccetti, 2000; Binner Bector et al., 2005; Al-Nimri and Bsoul, 2011). This means that ectopic eruption of maxillary first permanent molars, diagnosed at 6 to 7 years of age, may be a marker for the subsequent appearance of dental anomalies.

With the association between these tooth and developmental anomalies, it may be expected that in a sample of children with one of these anomalies, an increased frequency of the other associated anomalies would be found compared to the frequency found in the general population.

Infraocclusion of primary molars

The term infraocclusion describes a tooth or teeth, positioned below the occlusal plane, varying from 1 mm up to being embedded in the gingiva or in the alveolar bone. After normal eruption, some teeth start to be in infraocclusion and may show ankyloses (Figure 8.1).

Infraoccluded primary molars can be found in children as young as 3 to 4 years of age; however, it occurs most frequently at the age of 8 to 9 years. About 14% of children in this age group have one or more primary molars in infraocclusion. It is found twice as frequently in the mandible as in the maxilla, and the mandibular second primary molars are most affected. There is a genetic component to the anomaly, and in a group of siblings of children with infraocclusion, the prevalence of infraocclusion is higher (Kurol, 1981).

If primary molars show infraocclusion, it is very difficult or even impossible to move them into normal occlusion by orthodontic treatment. This contrasts with permanent molars, where it is sometimes possible, even in severe cases, to move the molar into occlusion again with orthodontic treatment (Figure 8.2).

Depending on the severity of the infraocclusion, there is a risk that tipping of adjacent permanent teeth will cause space loss for the permanent premolar.

In most cases with a permanent successor, the infraoccluded primary molars show progression of the infraocclusion. The exfoliation of the infraoccluded primary molars is normally delayed by about 6 months (Kurol and Thilander, 1984). However, the delay could also amount to 1 or 2 years, compared to contralateral teeth in the normal position.

An infraoccluded primary molar without a permanent successor is frequently associated with ankylosis. Percussion is a diagnostic tool for ankylosis using, for example, the handle of a metal mouth mirror. Ankylosed teeth typically have a solid sound when percussed, which is different from the sound heard when percussing a tooth suspended in a normal periodontal ligament (PDL).

In cases with agenesis of the permanent successor, a treatment plan is required already at the age of 9 to 10 years. In cases with severe infraocclusion at these ages, the infraocclusion is likely to worsen, and extraction of the primary molar is often the best solution. Later, orthodontic treatment is necessary to close the gaps and correct tipping of adjacent teeth; otherwise, a prosthetic treatment or transplantation of a maxillary third molar can be the solution.

If the primary molar is persisting at 12 to 14 years of age, without any severe infraocclusion or root resorption, there is good prognosis for long-term survival of the primary molar (Bjerklin and Bennett, 2000; Bjerklin et al., 2008).

Ectopic eruption of maxillary first permanent molar

The term 'ectopic eruption' describes a disturbance of the path of eruption, which causes a

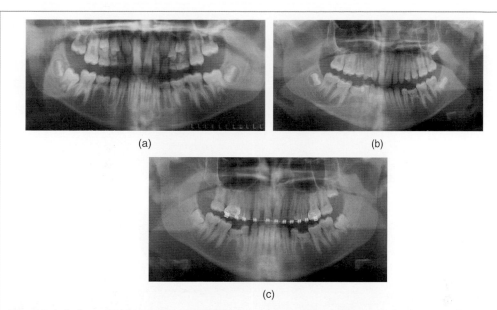

Figure 8.1 At the age of 11.6 years, the mandibular second primary molars are in occlusion, and there is agenesis of the mandibular second premolars (a). Two years later, infraocclusion is evident on both primary molars (b). At the age of 16, a more pronounced infraocclusion on the second primary molars and the first premolars have started to tip distally (c).

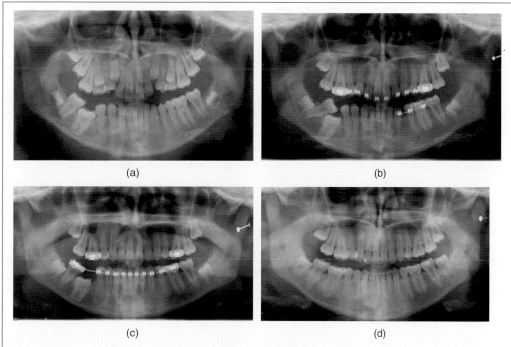

Figure 8.2 Severe infraocclusion of the mandibular right first permanent molar, age 12 (a). Further tipping of the adjacent teeth (b). Space gaining and surgical exposure of the infraoccluded permanent molar (c). After orthodontic traction, the molar has erupted into occlusion (d).

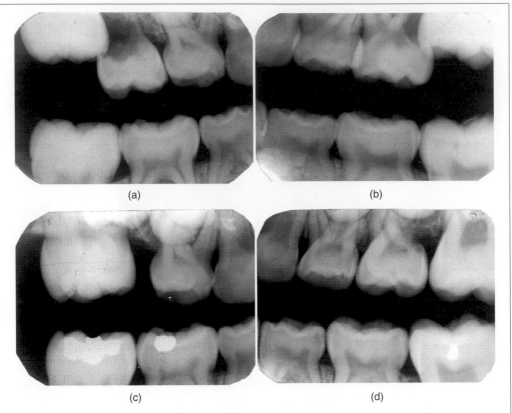

(a)

(b)

(c)

(d)

Figure 8.3 Girl, 6 years of age, maxillary first permanent molars in ectopic eruption and atypical resorption on the second primary molars (a,b). Right second primary molar is lost and severe space deficiency for the second premolar due to mesial movement of the first permanent molar (c). In (d), the left permanent molar has freed itself and shows reversible ectopic eruption.

tooth or teeth to erupt from their normal position, usually affecting maxillary first permanent molars and maxillary canines. The diagnosis can be made from panoramic, periapical or bitewing radiographs (Figure 8.3).

Ectopic eruption of maxillary first permanent molars occurs as a local eruption disturbance at the age of 6 to 7 years. The molar erupts in a mesial direction, resulting in a locked position, apical to the prominence on the distal surface of the second primary molar. There are two types, the reversible and the irreversible (Figure 8.3).

The reversible type is self-correcting. The permanent molar spontaneously frees itself and erupts into occlusion. The second primary molar remains in the mouth, with a variable amount of resorption of the distal aspect.

The irreversible type of ectopic eruption means that the permanent molar remains locked

in its position, above and distal to the primary molar, until the primary tooth is exfoliated or some type of treatment is provided. It is generally difficult to determine whether the problem is reversible or irreversible at the age of 7 years, and it may not be clear until some years later.

No clear answer is given in the literature regarding its aetiology, although various factors alone or in combination have been mentioned. However, the hereditary factor seems to be of importance. It has been shown that the frequency of ectopic eruption of the maxillary first permanent molar is much higher in the siblings of children with the anomaly than it is for the rest of the population. One study showed that the frequency among the siblings was 20% compared to 4.3% for the rest of the population (Kurol and Bjerklin, 1982a). The ratio between the reversible and the irreversible types was equivalent to that for the general population.

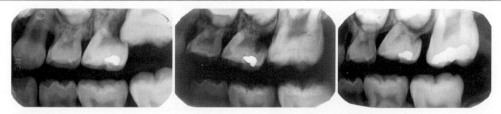

Figure 8.4 Left radiograph, girl, 7 years of age, with maxillary left permanent molar in ectopic eruption; the molar is still locked in the resorption distally on the second primary molar. Middle radiograph, 1 year later. The molar has freed itself, and the resorption is increased. Radiograph to the right shows the situation at the age of 9.5 years, with a hard tissue repair. In a follow-up study of 92 cases with resorbed second primary molar, 15 teeth showed hard tissue repair of the structure of the primary tooth, and this could be seen both on the radiographs and histologically (Kurol and Bjerklin, 1982a,1982b).

Treatment recommendation

In a young child with ectopic eruption of a maxillary first permanent molar, it is recommended to wait and evaluate whether the permanent molar will self correct spontaneously. If it becomes clear that the ectopic eruption is irreversible, and spontaneous correction does not occur, it is still recommended to postpone treatment until the second premolar is starting to erupt, because the primary molar should be retained as long as possible to hold the space. Even severely resorbed second primary molars will normally remain *in situ* until the normal exfoliation time (Figure 8.4) (Kurol and Bjerklin, 1982b; Bjerklin and Kurol, 1981). Most important is to advise the child and parents to keep the occlusal area of the permanent molar clean by showing correct brushing technique.

In cases where the second primary molar is lost, the consequences are mesial movement, tipping and rotation of the permanent molar. This may result in a loss of adequate space for the succeeding premolar (Mucedero *et al.*, 2015). Thus, depending on the amount of crowding that has arisen, these cases may require space gaining or extraction of permanent teeth. However, if the case is considered a non-extraction case, a space maintainer can be used to hold the space for the second premolar. In these cases, it is recommended to use a local space maintainer to avoid influencing the growth of the jaws. For instance, it is possible to place a band on the first permanent molar and a wire against the first primary molar (Figure 8.5).

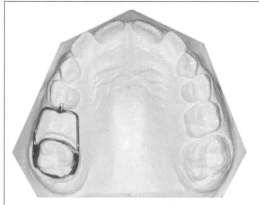

Figure 8.5 To avoid influencing growth of the jaw, a local space maintainer can be recommended in cases where space should be maintained until eruption of the second premolar.

Generally, when planning to correct ectopically erupted molars, it is important to consider that the correction shall be planned as part of the overall orthodontic therapy.

Attempting to release the maxillary molar by removing enamel and dentine from the distal aspect of the adjacent maxillary second primary molar tooth or releasing the maxillary molar by extraction of the maxillary second primary molar normally leads to further mesial positioning and angulation of the first permanent molar, with a risk that it will come into a poor occlusion, with severe mesial tipping and rotation.

Impacted maxillary canines

Impacted teeth are almost always in ectopic positions. Apart from third molars, maxillary

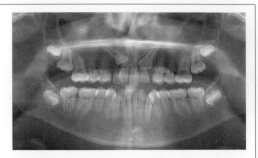

Figure 8.6 Both maxillary canines are impacted, and 3 of the maxillary incisors are resorbed.

canines are the teeth with the highest incidence of impaction. The frequency of impacted maxillary canines is 2 to 3% (Dachi and Howell, 1961; Thilander and Myrberg, 1973), and about 50% of them cause resorption on adjacent incisor roots. In 50 to 60% of such cases, the resorptions reach the pulp (Figure 8.6).

Impaction of maxillary permanent canines is a frequent clinical problem. The exact cause of impaction or ectopic canine eruption remains obscure. Along with the 'eruption path' theory, lack of space has been suggested as a causative factor, especially with labial impaction.

Along with the maxillary first permanent molar, a correctly positioned maxillary permanent canine is an important component of the dentition. It is an essential tooth for good occlusion because of its anatomy and position in the dental arch for proper function. Correct positioning is also required for good aesthetics.

The normal eruption path for the maxillary canine is with its crown directed mesially and somewhat palatally. It starts its eruption high up in the maxilla and moves towards the occlusal plane, gradually uprighting itself until it appears to strike the distal aspect of the root of the lateral incisor. It then seems to be deflected to a more vertical position, and it finally erupts with a slight mesial inclination. At the end of the eruption, it moves the incisors towards the midline. Broadbent (1941) suggests that displacement of the permanent maxillary canine is due to this long and tortuous eruption path. The permanent canine takes almost twice as long to erupt as the first permanent molar.

Early management

During the clinical assessment of 9- to 11-year-old children, there is an opportunity to prevent later problems, and this can be called 'early management'. The general dentist has to check the development of the dentition and ensure that normal canine eruption is occurring. The first step is palpation apical to the primary canine. The following clinical signs may be indications of an ectopically positioned canine or impaction:

■ absence of a normal labial canine bulge or a marked difference in the canine bulge between the right and the left sides at the palpation;
■ presence of a palatal bulge;
■ delayed eruption of a permanent canine or prolonged retention of a primary canine;
■ distal tipping or migration of the lateral incisor;
■ a widened canine dental follicle, as seen on periapical intra oral radiographs.

In 7 to 10% of children, the clinical investigation will need to be supplemented with intra oral or panoramic radiographs which, on average, means 2 or 3 children in a school class of 25 children.

Intervention will often require the extraction of primary canines (Figure 8.7), sometimes followed by limited appliance therapy (Ericson and Kurol, 1988; Armi *et al.*, 2011; Baccetti *et al.*, 2011). The eruptive direction of the permanent canine should improve within 12 months of the extraction of the primary canine; otherwise, it can be assumed that the permanent canine will not self-correct.

Late management situations

When it becomes clear that a canine is irreversibly impacted, there is normally a need to start treatment immediately. This group normally includes patients of 11 years or older in late mixed dentition or early permanent dentition, where intervention was not attempted for some reason or where extraction of the primary canines did not lead to an improvement in the eruption direction in the following 6 to 12 months. Also included will be cases with

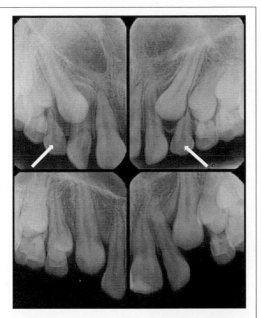

Figure 8.7 After extraction of primary canines (arrows point to the extracted primary canines). A favourable change in eruptive pathway was seen, leading to uneventful eruption.

atypical early root resorption on one or both adjacent incisors.

An overall orthodontic treatment plan will be required in these patients, since if there is suspicion of serious resorption of roots of the adjacent central and/or lateral incisors, it is important to produce an overall orthodontic treatment plan. This can include treatment to create space between the canine and the incisor root to prevent further resorption. In these cases, the long-term prognosis for the resorbed incisors is good (Becker and Chaushu, 2005; Bjerklin and Guitirokh, 2011).

Furthermore, the later management cases require sophisticated evaluations, often involving tomography. Computed tomography improves the accuracy of location of impacted maxillary canines and resorption status of adjacent roots (Figure 8.8), thus allowing better treatment planning for both surgical and orthodontic treatments (Oberoi and Kneuppel, 2012). Only about 50% of the resorptions on the palatal or buccal aspects of incisor roots can be detected by intra oral or panoramic radiographs (Ericson and Kurol, 2000; Walker *et al.*, 2005).

One of the main issues to consider when drawing up a treatment plan for patients with impacted maxillary canines is whether root resorption is present on the adjacent lateral or central incisors. Using this information, a decision can be made about the best time to start treatment; patients in this group normally need surgical exposure of the impacted canines and a long and complex orthodontic treatment.

Canine dental follicle

There is no evidence for treatment because of a large follicle. The dental follicles of impacted maxillary canines are normally enlarged (Ericson and Bjerklin, 2001), and the anatomical structures close to the follicles have an influence on its width and form. A widened follicle of a maxillary canine is a sign of ectopic position or impaction of the canine, especially when the canine is palatally displaced.

The follicles are often seen to expand into the soft cancellous bone close to, and sometimes around, the roots of the adjacent permanent teeth (Figure 8.9).

It is sometimes claimed in the literature that an enlarged dental follicle of an impacted maxillary canine can cause root resorption on the neighbouring incisor and that there is a risk for cystic degeneration, but there is no evidence to confirm this; rather, the opposite has been shown (Ericson *et al.*, 2002).

The assessment of root resorption and canine position

The normal orthodontic assessment will be needed to evaluate the malocclusion and decide whether the case requires extraction of permanent teeth. Without CBCT in extraction cases, there is a high risk of leaving severely resorbed incisors and extracting healthy premolars (Bjerklin and Ericson, 2006).

If there is a need to extract a root resorbed lateral incisor, a decision will be required about whether to also extract the other lateral incisor for symmetry.

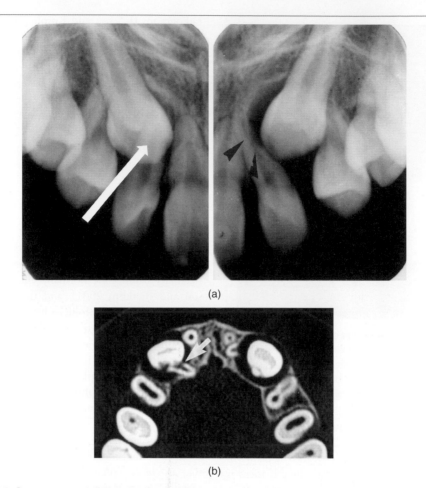

(a)

(b)

Figure 8.8 Severe space deficiency in the maxilla and ectopic position of the two maxillary canines (a). It is not possible to diagnose any root resorption on the right lateral incisor (white arrow). In (b), the CT slice shows severe root resorption on both the lateral incisors.

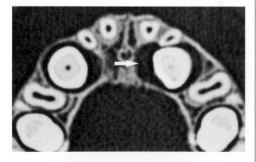

Figure 8.9 Maxillary right canine in a normal eruption and position. The left canine in ectopic position palatally displaced with a widened follicle (white arrow).

Orthodontic treatment of impacted maxillary canines after surgical exposure

At the start of the treatment, it is important to know whether there are root resorptions on the adjacent teeth. When there are resorptions or a high probability of resorptions, the canine must be moved away from the incisor first, before starting the traction out towards the alveolar crest. This can be done in different ways. One method is to start with a transpalatal arch for anchorage and place heavy wires soldered to the bands. These wires can be 0.8 or 0.9 mm in diameter and provided with eyelets. With this appliance, it is easy to change the direction of the

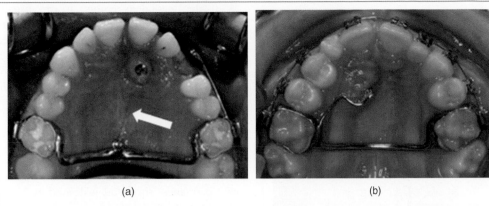

(a)   (b)

Figure 8.10 In (a), a case with a slight resorption of the maxillary left central incisor root. Orthodontic traction (white arrow) of the left canine away from the incisor root after surgical open exposure. In (b), with aid of a sectional arch, the canine is moved away from the incisor root after surgical closed exposure.

traction with the elastic thread. These wires can be placed on one or both sides of the bands to get the best possible choice of traction direction. If distal movement is needed, a loop can be soldered directly onto the transpalatal arch, or after open exposure, an elastic thread can be placed directly onto the canine (Figure 8.10).

For some patients, all the maxillary teeth can be bonded or bracketed at the start of the treatment. When the case reaches heavier working wires, the canine can be moved towards the labial wire using elastic forces. This approach is more suitable for non-extraction cases, where there is a need to regain space for the canine and where the ectopic position is not severe.

If the ectopic maxillary canine can be distanced from the root of an incisor which is showing damage, the resorption process will cease. The affected tooth will not be susceptible to further damage, and the risk for increased mobility or discoloration is minimal.

Supernumerary teeth

Supernumerary teeth are often in the form of a mesiodens between the maxillary central incisors and may lead to delayed eruption or impaction of maxillary incisors.

Delayed eruption may also be caused by premature loss of primary incisors due to trauma, which often is followed by a fibrotic gingiva, or early loss of a primary incisor.

Furthermore, delayed eruption of maxillary incisors can be caused by odontogenic tumours

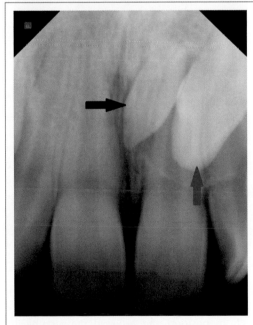

Figure 8.11 A peg-shaped mesiodens (black arrow) and an impacted canine (blue arrow).

such as odontomas and cysts, but these conditions are very rare.

Mesiodens

Normally the mesiodentes are discovered at the ages of 7 to 9 years. Often, a mesiodens is palatally positioned and can be in an upside-down position with the root between the roots of the central incisors and with its crown

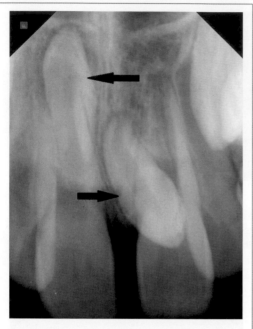

Figure 8.12 In cases with two mesiodentes (black arrows), the crowns are most often positioned in different directions. About 25% of the patients with mesiodens have two mesiodentes.

apical to the central incisor's root apices. Most mesiodentes have a conical or peg-shape crown anatomy (Figure 8.11). When there are two mesiodentes, they often are positioned with the crowns in different directions (Figure 8.12).

Almost 50% of the mesiodentes have resorptions, but complications such as resorption of adjacent teeth or cyst formation because of a mesiodens are rare (Mensah *et al.*, 2015).

Mesiodentes, which do not interfere with erupting teeth or occlusal development, can be left in position and followed radiographically every second year during the growth period of the jaws, and further radiographic follow-ups are not indicated.

If the mesiodens erupts, it can usually be removed without problems. On the other hand, in a patient who has a palatal positioned mesiodens and active orthodontic treatment is considered, for example for space closure or proclination of the maxillary incisors, removal of the mesiodens may be necessary.

Conclusions

The exfoliation of infraoccluded primary molars with permanent successors is delayed by 1 to 2 years compared to contralateral teeth in normal positions.

Ectopic eruption of maxillary first permanent molars has a clear hereditary factor. The prognosis for the atypically resorbed second primary molars is good; therefore, it is important to avoid any type of treatment to release the permanent molar from the resorption cavity of the second primary molar.

About 50% of the impacted maxillary canines cause resorption on the adjacent incisor roots. At the ages of 9 to 11 years, the permanent maxillary canines should be palpable buccally above the primary canines, and if not palpable, radiographic examination should be performed.

In children with palatally displaced maxillary canines and no signs of root resorptions on the adjacent incisors, the first option is to remove the primary canines. An improved eruption direction should be evident within a 12-month period; otherwise, orthodontic treatment must be incorporated to move the canine into the correct position.

A mesiodens that does not interfere with adjacent erupting teeth or occlusal development can be left in the jaw without treatment.

REFERENCES

Al-Nimri, K. and Bsoul, E. (2011) Maxillary palatal canine impaction displacement in subjects with congenitally missing maxillary lateral incisors. Am J Orthod Dentofacial Orthop 140: 81–86.

Armi, P., Cozza, P. and Baccetti, T. (2011) Effect of RME and headgear treatment on the eruption of palatally displaced canines. A randomized clinical study. Angle Orthod. 81: 370–374.

Baccetti, T. (2000) Tooth anomalies associated with failure of eruption of first and second permanent molars. Am J Orthod Dentofacial Orthop 118: 608–610.

Baccetti, T., Sigler, L.M. and McNamara, Jr. J.A. (2011) A RCT on treatment of palatally displaced canines with RME and/or a transpalatal arch. Eur J Orthod 33: 601–607.

Becker, A. and Chaushu, S. (2005) Long-term follow-up of severely resorbed maxillary incisors after resolution of an etiologically associated impacted canine. Am J Orthod Dentofacial Orthop 127: 650–654.

Binner Becktor, K., Steiniche, K. and Kjær, I. (2005) Association between ectopic eruption of maxillary canines and first molars. Eur J Orthod 27: 186–189.

Bjerklin, K., Kurol, J. and Valentine, J. (1992) Ectopic eruption of maxillary first permanent molars and association with other tooth and developmental disturbances. Eur J Orthod 14: 369–375.

Bjerklin, K. and Bennett, J. (2000) The long-term survival of lower second primary molars in subjects with agenesis of the premolars. Eur J Orthod 22: 245–255.

Bjerklin, K. and Ericson, S. (2006) How a computerized tomography examination changed the treatment plans of 80 children with retained and ectopically positioned maxillary canines. Angle Orthod 76: 43–51.

Bjerklin, K. and Guitirokh, C.H. (2011) Maxillary incisor root resorption induced by ectopic canines. A follow-up study, 13 to 28 years posttreatment. Angle Orthod 1–7.

Bjerklin, K. and Kurol, J. (1981) Prevalence of ectopic eruption of the maxillary first permanent molar. Swed Dent J 5: 29–34.

Bjerklin, K., Kurol, J. and Valentine, J. (1992) Ectopic eruption of maxillary first permanent molars and association with other tooth and developmental disturbances. Eur J Orthod 14: 369–375.

Bjerklin, K., Al-Najjar, M., Kårestedt, H. et al. (2008) Agenesis of mandibular second premolars with retained primary molars. A longitudinal radiographic study of 99 subjects from 12 years of age to adulthood. Eur J Orthod 30: 254–261.

Broadbent, B.H. (1941) Ontogenic development of occlusion. Angle Orthod 11: 223–241.

Dachi, S.F. and Howell, F.V. (1961) A survey of 3,874 routine full mouth radiographs. Oral Surg Oral Med Oral Path 14: 1165–1169.

Ericson, S. and Kurol, J. (1988) Early treatment of palatally erupting maxillary canines by extraction of the primary canines. Eur J Orthod 10: 283–295.

Ericson, S. and Bjerklin, K. (2001) The dental follicle in normally and ectopically erupting maxillary canines: a computed tomography study. Angle Orthod 71: 333–342.

Ericson, S. and Kurol, J. (2000) Resorption of incisors after ectopic eruption of maxillary canines: a CT study. Angle Orthod 70: 415–423.

Ericson, S., Bjerklin, K. and Falahat, B. (2002) Does the canine dental follicle cause resorption of permanent incisor roots? A computed tomographic study of erupting maxillary canines. Angle Orthod 72: 95–104.

Hoffmeister, H. (1977) Mikrosymptome als Hinweis auf vererbte Unterzahl, Überzahl und Verlagerung von Zähnen. Deutsche Zahnärztliche Zeitung 32: 551–561.

Kurol, J. (1981) Infraocclusion of primary molars: an epidemiologic and familial study. Community Dent Oral Epidemiol 9: 94–102.

Kurol, J. and Bjerklin, K. (1982a) Ectopic eruption of maxillary first permanent molars: familial tendencies. J Dent Child 49: 35–38.

Kurol, J. and Bjerklin, K. (1982b) Resorption of maxillary second primary molars caused by ectopic eruption of the maxillary first permanent molar: a longitudinal and histological study. J Dent Child 4: 273–279.

Kurol, J. and Thilander, B. (1984) Infraocclusion of primary molars and the effect on occlusal development: a longitudinal study. Eur J Orthod 6: 277–293.

Mensah T, Garvald H, Grindefjord, M. *et al.* (2015) Idiopathic resorption of impacted mesiodentes: a radiographic study. Eur Arch Paediatr Dent. doi 10.1007/s40368-014-0162-8.

Mucedero, M., Rozzi, M., Cardoni, G. *et al.* (2015) Dentoskeletal features in individuals with ectopic eruption of the permanent maxillary first molar. Korean J Orthod 45: 190–196.

Oberoi, S. and Kneuppel, S. (2012) Three-dimensional assessment of impacted canines and root resorption using cone beam computed tomography. Oral Surg Oral Med Oral Pathol Oral Radiol Endod 113: 260–267.

Pfeifer, G. (1974) Systematik und Morphologie der kraniofazialen Anomalien. In: *Fortschritte der Kiefer – und Gesichts – Chirurgie Bd* (Ed. K. Schuchardt), 18. Stuttgardt: Georg Thieme Verlag, pp. 1–14.

Thilander, B. and Myrberg, N. (1973) The prevalence of malocclusion in Swedish school children. Scand J Dent Res 81: 12–20.

Walker, L., Enciso, R. and Mah, J. (2005) Three-dimensional localization of maxillary canines with cone-beam computed tomography. Am J Orthod Dentofacial Orthop 128: 418–423.

PART 3

Tissue Response to Orthodontic and Orthopaedic Forces

Despite differences in design of removable and fixed appliances, all of them are acting, by orthodontic or orthopaedic forces, on teeth and adjacent structures as well as on condyles and facial sutures.

An optimal force intends to induce a maximal cellular response and stability of the tissue, whereas an unfavourable one may initiate adverse tissue reactions.

Retention is the stable phase of the orthodontic procedure, and is of importance for the post-retention outcome.

Essential Orthodontics, First Edition. Birgit Thilander, Krister Bjerklin and Lars Bondemark.
© 2018 John Wiley & Sons Ltd. Published 2018 by John Wiley & Sons Ltd.

CHAPTER 9

Tissue response to orthodontic forces

Brigit Thilander

Key topics

- Tooth-supporting tissues
- Physiologic tooth migration
- Orthodontic tooth movements
- Transmission of orthodontic forces into cellular reactions
- Biomechanical principles

Learning objectives

- To understand the sense of physiological tooth migration in orthodontics
- To understand and describe the hyaline phase in tooth movements
- To understand and describe the tissue reaction on the pressure and tension sides in orthodontic tooth movements
- To understand the transmission of orthodontic forces into cellular reactions
- To describe the tissue reaction in the different kinds of tooth movements

Essential Orthodontics, First Edition. Birgit Thilander, Krister Bjerklin and Lars Bondemark.
© 2018 John Wiley & Sons Ltd. Published 2018 by John Wiley & Sons Ltd.

Introduction

Orthodontic treatment comprises a wealth of removable and fixed appliances. Despite differences in design, they all involve the use and control of forces acting on the teeth and adjacent structures. Changes from such forces are seen in the dentoalveolar system, resulting in tooth movements, opposite to the forces that have an influence on sutures and condyles by means of dentofacial orthopaedics (Chapter 10). An optimal orthodontic force intends to induce a maximal cellular response and to establish stability of the tissue, whereas an unfavourable one may initiate adverse tissue reactions (Chapter 11). The purpose of this chapter is to focus on tissue reactions in the periodontium during the active phase of orthodontic treatment, while those during the retention and post-retention periods will be described in Chapter 12.

Tooth-supporting tissues

Tooth movement is a complicated process, requiring changes in the gingiva, periodontal ligament (PDL), root cementum, and alveolar bone with their differences in cell population and remodelling capacity. Therefore, a brief description of the normal periodontium is given.

Gingiva

The predominant component of the gingiva is the connective tissue, which consists of collagen fibres, fibroblasts, nerves and matrix. Fibroblasts are engaged in the production of various types of fibres, but are also involved in the synthesis of the connective tissue matrix. Collagen fibres are bundles of collagen fibrils with distinct orientation and divided into circular, dentogingival, dentoperiosteal and trans-septal fibres, and provide the resilience for maintaining the architectural form of the dentogingival attachment.

Periodontal ligament

The periodontal ligament (PDL), about 0.25 mm wide, is the soft, richly vascular and cellular connective tissue that surrounds the roots of the teeth and joins the root cementum with the alveolar bone. The true periodontal fibres, principal fibres, develop along with the

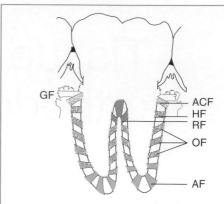

Figure 9.1 The PDL fibres: alveolar-crest fibres (ACF), apical fibres (AF), gingival fibres (GF), horizontal fibres (HF), oblique fibres (OF) and interradicular fibres (RF).

eruption of the tooth, and their orientation alters continuously during tooth eruption. When the tooth has reached contact in occlusion, they constitute the following well-oriented groups (Figure 9.1): alveolar crest fibres and horizontal, oblique, apical, and inter-radicular fibres. The individual bundles have a slightly wavy course, which allows the tooth to move within its socket (physiologic mobility). The presence of a PDL is essential for tooth movements in orthodontic treatment.

The fibrils are embedded in a ground substance with connective tissue polysaccharides (glycosaminoglycans), which vary with age. The tissue response to orthodontic forces, including cell mobilization and conversion of collagen fibres, is considerably slower in older individuals than in children and adolescents. During physiological conditions, collagen turnover in PDL is much higher than that in most other tissues (e.g. twice as high as that of the gingiva). The high turnover has been attributed to the fact that forces on the PDL are multidirectional, having vertical and horizontal components. The lower collagen turnover in the gingiva may result from the lowered functional stress as the trans-septal fibres function in a manner similar to tendons, providing firm anchorage of the tooth.

Root cementum

The cementum is a specialized tissue covering the root surface. It contains no blood vessels, has

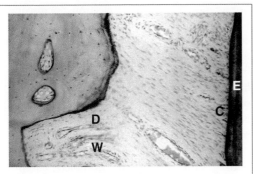

Figure 9.2 Area from a 22-year-old patient. Chain of cementoblasts (C) along a thick layer of cementum. Widened capillary in a cleft, where bone resorption may start during the initial stage of tooth movement (W). Darkly stained surface line containing connective tissue polysaccharides (D) and note the absence of osteoblasts along the bone surface. Embedded principal fibres in the cementum of the tooth (E).

no innervation, does not undergo remodelling, and is characterized by continuing deposition throughout life. During root formation, a primary cementum is formed. After tooth eruption and in response to functional demands, a secondary cementum is formed that, in contrast to the primary cementum, contain cells. During the continuous formation of the primary cementum, portions of the principle fibres in the PDL adjacent to the root become imbedded and mineralized (Figure 9.2).

Alveolar bone

The alveolar process forms and supports the sockets of the teeth and consists of dense outer cortical bone plates with varying amounts of spongy or cancellous bone between them. The thickness of the cortical laminae varies in different locations. The cancellous bone contains bone trabeculae, the architecture of which is partly genetically determined and partly the result of forces to which teeth are exposed during function or orthodontic treatment. The type of bone through which the tooth is displaced should be considered in the orthodontic treatment plan. Tooth movements in a mesial or distal direction displace the roots through the cancellous bone with its rapid remodelling capacity, in contrast to tooth movements labially

or lingually into the thin cortical plates with risk of bony defects.

Physiologic tooth migration

Tissue reactions in the tooth-supporting tissues are connected not only with orthodontic treatment but also with eruption of the teeth and development of the occlusion. The teeth and their supporting tissues have a life-long ability to adapt to functional demands and hence drift through the alveolar process, a phenomenon called physiologic tooth migration. When the teeth migrate, they bring the supra-alveolar fibres with them, which means remodelling of the PDL and alveolar bone, as illustrated in Figure 9.3. Osteoclasts, associated with the resorptive surface, are seen along the bone wall, towards which the tooth is migrating, while osteoblasts are seen at the bone wall, from which it is moving away (depository side).

Because considerable changes in tooth position occur without any orthodontic intervention, knowledge of periodontal remodelling during physiologic tooth migration is of utmost importance when evaluating the long-term effects of an orthodontic treatment.

Orthodontic tooth movements

Basically, no great difference exists between the tissue reactions observed in physiologic tooth

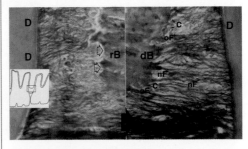

Figure 9.3 Physiologic migration in the rat in the interdental area in direction of the black arrow. Resorptive alveolar bone surface (rB, and at open arrows). Depository alveolar bone surface (dB). Older fibres (oF) included in the new bone formation by osteoclasts. New fibrils (nF) near the bone surface and in the middle of the PDL. Osteoblasts (C) and dentin (D).

migration and those observed in orthodontic tooth movements. Because the teeth are moved more rapidly during treatment, the tissue changes elicited by orthodontic forces are more significant and extensive. Application of a force on the crown of the tooth leads to a response in its surrounding tissue, resulting in an orthodontic tooth movement. Already in 1904, Carl Sandstedt's studies in dogs demonstrated that tooth movement is a process of resorption at the 'pressure side' and deposition of bone at the 'tension side' (Sandstedt, 1904). He gave the first description of the glasslike appearance of the compressed tissue, called hyalinisation, which has been associated with a standstill of the tooth movement. But it was not until 1951 that tooth movements attracted wider attention with Kaare Reitan's classic study 'The initial tissue reaction incident to orthodontic tooth movement'. He used the dog as an experimental model but also extracted teeth from humans, and histology was his means to address the questions of clinical importance. By means of electron microscopy, Rygh (1972) continued Reitan's research. Rygh could explain why orthodontic tooth movements might cause damage to the tooth, probably as a sequel of the hyalinisation process. They have been my co-authors in some textbooks, and some of their unique histological material has been used even in the present chapter, by permission of Elsevier Publishers.

Our knowledge of the reactions of the supporting structures is still incomplete. From a clinical point of view it is, however, known that the initial tooth movement is followed by a stop, due to hyalinisation, whereupon the movement will continue.

Initial phase of tooth movement

Application of a force to the crown of a tooth leads to tooth movement within the alveolus and initially a narrowing of the PDL, causing compression in limited areas and by that

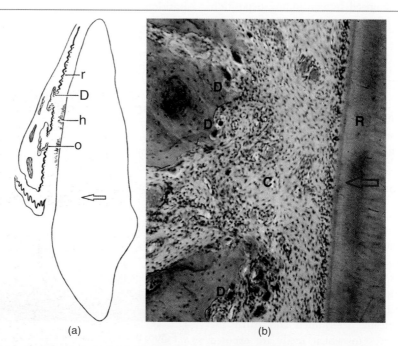

(a)　　　　　　　　　(b)

Figure 9.4 In the drawing to the left (a), location of bone resorption adjacent to the apical third of a maxillary canine. The tooth was moved continuously for 3 weeks. Compensatory formation of osteoid in open marrow spaces (o) and remnants of hyalinised tissue adhering to the root surface (h). Direct bone resorption adjacent to the apical third of the root (D). In (b) to the right, direct resorption with osteoclasts along the bone surface (D) and absence of epithelial remnants in adjacent periodontal tissue, i.e. centre of the formerly cell-free zone (C). The tooth root (R), and the blue arrows show the force and tooth movement direction.

impedes vascular circulation and cell differentiation (Rygh, 1972). Advanced cellular and vascular changes may occur within a few hours of the application of the orthodontic force (Rygh, 1973). The cells undergo a series of changes, starting with a swelling of the mitochondria and the endoplasmatic reticulum, and continuing with rupture and dissolution of the cell membrane. This leaves only isolated nuclei between compressed fibrous elements (pyknosis) and is the first indication of hyalinisation. Precursor cells along the alveolar bone wall differentiate into osteoclasts and fibroblasts in young humans after 30 to 40 hours (Reitan, 1951).

Hyalinisation phase

At the pressure side, the degradation of the cells and vascular structures gives the tissue a glasslike appearance under the light microscope, termed hyalinisation (Figure 9.4). It is caused partly by anatomic and partly by mechanical factors and is almost unavoidable in clinical orthodontics. Hyalinization represents a sterile necrotic area, characterized by three main stages: degeneration, elimination of destroyed tissue, and establishment of a new tooth attachment.

Degeneration starts where the pressure is highest and the narrowing of the PDL is most obvious, that is, around the bone spicules. In the hyalinised zones, there are no cells that can differentiate into osteoclasts, since osteoclast precursor cells cannot enter from the compressed and degenerated blood vessels. Therefore, no direct resorption of the bone surface at the PDL side can take place. Instead, the osteoclasts are formed and start the resorption from the alveolar bone marrow spaces (undermining bone resorption) (Figure 9.5). After the initial phase of tooth movement, the process stops until the adjacent alveolar bone has been removed by undermining osteoclastic bone resorption. The necrotic structures are removed, and the hyalinised area repopulated by cells. A limited hyalinised zone may persist from 3 to 4 weeks in a young patient, while its duration is longer in adults.

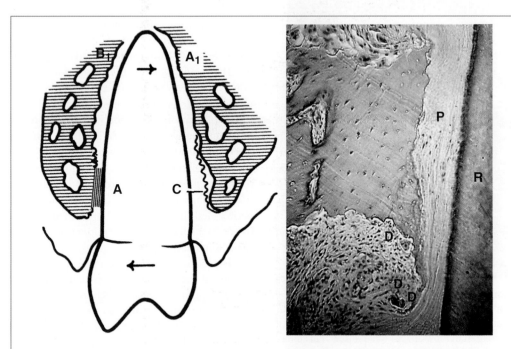

Figure 9.5 To the left, in most cases, tooth movement is initiated by formation of a cell-free area (A) and new osteoid at (C). The pressure site (A1) and tension site (B1). To the right, a maxillary first premolar in a 12-year-old patient represents the area A in the figure to the left. Root surface (R) and remaining pyknotic cell nuclei in hyalinised tissue (P). Direct bone resorption with osteoclasts (D).

The peripheral areas of the hyalinised compressed tissue are eliminated by an invasion of cells and blood vessels from the undamaged PDL (Rygh, 1973). The hyalinised tissue is ingested by the phagocytic activity of macrophages and is removed completely and the re-establishment will start (Brudvik and Rygh, 1994).

Root resorption

A side effect of the cellular activity during the removal of the necrotic hyalinised tissue is that the cementoid layer of the root is left with a raw unprotected surface, which readily can be attacked by resorptive cells (Brudvik and Rygh, 1994). Root resorption then occurs around this cell-free tissue, starting at the border of the hyalinised zone (Figure 9.6) (Brudvik and Rygh, 1993). The first sign of resorption (initial phase) was defined as a penetration of cells

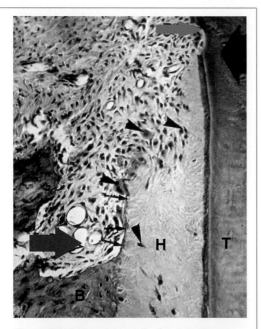

Figure 9.6 Photomicrograph of the hyalinised zone (H) between alveolar bone (B) and root surface of the tooth (T). Alveolar bone resorption occurs from marrow spaces (blue arrow) and small arrows indicate thin line of bone between the resorbed bone and hyaline tissue. Small amount of root resorption (green arrow) at the border of the hyaline zone (adapted from Brudvik and Rygh, 1993).

from the periphery of the necrotic tissue, where mononucleated fibroblast-like cells started removing the precementum at the cementum surface. Beneath the main hyalinised zone, resorption of the outer layer of the cementum occurred in a later phase, during which multi-nucleated phagocytes were involved in removing the main mass of necrotic PDL tissue (Figure 9.7). Repair of the lacunae occurs after termination of force and in absence of necrotic tissue (Brudvik and Rygh, 1995) (Figure 9.8). The first sign was a synthesis of collagenous fibrillary material by fibroblast-like cells, followed by re-establishment of the new PDL. Further studies are needed, however, to fully clarify the factors leading to transition of an active process of root resorption into one of repair.

Secondary phase of tooth movement

The PDL space is now wider than before the start of the treatment and the tissue under repair is rich in cells. On the pressure side, the osteoclastic bone resorption continues with a predominantly direct bone resorption, as long as the force is kept within certain limits or gentle reactivation (Figure 9.9). With a favourable force, the tooth movement is rapid.

The main feature is the deposition of new bone on the alveolar surface from which the tooth is moving (the tension side) (Figure 9.10). Cell proliferation usually occurs after 30 to 40 hours in young humans. A 'pre-bone' protein matrix, or osteoid, is produced by osteoblasts on the tension side. The formation of this new osteoid is related to the form and thickness of the fibre bundles in the PDL. The originally periodontal fibres become embedded in the osteoid, which continuously mineralises to bone tissue in its deeper layer.

The bone deposition on the periodontal surface on the tension side is synchronous with the resorption process, which occurs on the pressure side of the alveolar bone and tends to maintain the dimension of the supporting bone tissue. Extensive remodelling takes place in the deeper cell-rich layers of the periosteum, a reaction that tends to restore the thickness of the supporting bone.

The observation that orthodontic tooth movement involves many inflammation-like

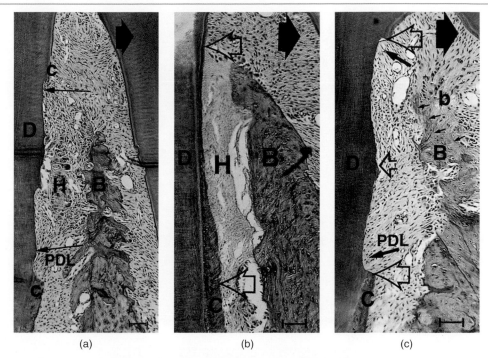

(a)   (b)   (c)

Figure 9.7 Photomicrographs of the root resorption and repair sequence of the compressed PDL 21 days after tooth movement in the direction of the black arrows. Cementum (C), dentin (D) and hyalinised zone (H). To the left (a), neighbouring section with repair of peripheral parts of resorption lacunae by deposition cementum (thin arrows). In the middle (b), the length of the hyalinised zone (between the two open arrows) after 3 days of compression. To the right (c), the length of root resorption (between the two open arrows) after 21 days of tooth movement. Note the regular arrangement of the PDL cells and fibres in the peripheral part of the resorption lacunae (medium arrows). In the central part of resorption area (small open arrow), no trace of fibres is connected with the root surface. The small black arrows show the demarcation line between old bone (B) and new bond (b) in crest area (adapted from Brudvik and Rygh, 1995).

reactions at the pressure side is to be understood as a response to the orthodontic forces. The term inflammation should not be confused with the term infection, as is often the case in popular use. In orthodontics, this inflammatory process is occurring in a local environment as a cellular response to a force that is transiently causing tissue degeneration.

Transmission of orthodontic forces into cellular reactions

The orthodontic tooth movement is initiated by mechanical forces. However, the transmission of the orthodontic force to a biological response in the periodontal tissues is not related to the mechanic sensing by the osteocytes, as in the bone remodelling sequence (see Chapter 3).

The accepted concept today is that an aseptic inflammation is the initiating factor for tooth movement. This is in line with histological studies described above, demonstrating necrotic/hyaline areas, vasodilatation, and migration of leucocytes from the blood vessels, i.e. tissue degeneration with an inflammatory reaction, which promotes the tissue reactions and bone resorption at compression sites.

Inflammatory mediators including cytokines, for example interleukins (IL-1, IL-6, tumour necrosis factors (TNF-a), neuropeptides, and prostaglandins (PG) are produced in the PDL (Ransjö *et al.*, 1998; Meikle, 2006; Wise and King, 2008). Immunohistochemical staining has confirmed the localisation of pro-inflammatory mediators in periodontal tissues in response to orthodontic forces

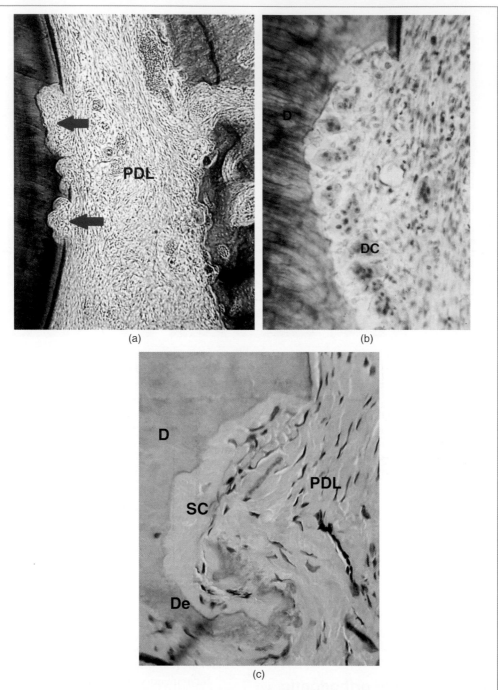

(a)

(b)

(c)

Figure 9.8 To the left (a), superficial root resorption (blue arrows). In (b), magnification of the root resorption area in the figure to the left. Dentin (D) and dentinoclasts (DC). In (c), repaired lacuna with demarcation (De), secondary cementum (SC), dentin (D) and periodontal ligament (PDL).

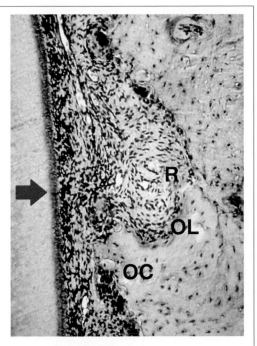

Figure 9.9 Effect on pressure side of a maxillary premolar of a 12-year-old. The tooth is moved as indicated by the blue arrow. An osteoid layer that persists (OL) bordered the alveolar bone. Extensive bone resorption (R) has occurred in the area subjacent to this osteoid tissue. The bone surface is lined with osteoclasts (OC).

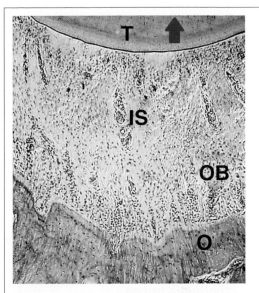

Figure 9.10 Effect of a force of 45 cN during 36 hours on the tension side of a second incisor. The tooth is moved as indicated by the blue arrow. Note the increase and spreading of new cells in areas close to the bone surface and to the stretched fibre bundles. Tooth root (T), interstitial space (IS) proliferating osteoblasts (OB) between fibre bundles and increase osteoid tissue (O).

(Davidovitch *et al.,* 1988). The important role of PGs as a mediator of the tissue response to the mechanical force is demonstrated by inhibition of orthodontic tooth movement in experimental animals with systemic or local administration of PG inhibitors.

The inflammatory mediators will bind to specific receptors on target cells and start an intracellular signalling cascade increasing second messengers (e.g. cAMP and Ca^{2+}) and activation of gene transcription factors. This will ultimately lead to changes in cell differentiation and altered functions. Moreover, in response to the orthodontic force and the increased levels of inflammatory mediators, there is an up-regulation of receptor activator of nuclear factor kappa-B ligand (RANKL) expression in cells at the compression sites. RANKL binds to the receptor RANK on osteoclast precursors and leads to an increase in formation and activation of osteoclasts, and subsequently an increase

in bone resorption. The RANKL/RANK/OPG system is thus an important part, not only in bone remodelling and tooth eruption, but also in orthodontic tooth movements (Wise and King, 2008).

The mechanisms at the tension site, leading to increased formation of alveolar bone and remodelling of the PDL, is not fully understood. The mechanical force, leading to a strain in the tissue, will affect cellular interactions with adjacent cells and adhesion to matrix proteins via membrane proteins. This will alter the gene expression in the target cells and change cellular activities, although the precise molecular mechanisms are unknown. The anabolic effect and the stimulated bone formation at the tension site can be compared to the osteogenic response in sutures in clinical treatments with maxillary suture expansion and osteo-distraction.

Although orthodontic tooth movement is a local process within the jawbones, systemic effects on the skeleton will probably interact with the biological process. Taken together, endocrine and metabolic interactions involving the skeleton, of which the craniofacial bones are integrated parts, may have implications for the orthodontic treatment in patients with metabolic diseases and related pharmacological medication.

Biomechanical principles

Application of a force on the crown of the tooth results in tooth movement, which depends on type, magnitude, direction and duration of the force. The biological process in the tissue response is of fundamental significance in making the proper use of all these biomechanical principles.

Orthodontic forces

Two different types of orthodonitic forces exist: continuous and intermittent. Modern fixed appliance systems are based on light continuous forces from an arch-wire. However, a continuous force may be interrupted after a limited period, when it is no longer active and has to be reactivated. Such an interrupted continuous force has certain advantages in clinical orthodontics, as the tissues are given ample time for reorganization, which is favourable for further tissue changes when the force is again activated. An intermittent force acts during a short period and is induced primarily by removable functional appliances.

The magnitude of forces is important for the tissue response. A light force over a certain distance moves a tooth more rapidly and with fewer injuries to the supporting tissues than a heavy force (Reitan, 1964; Owman-Moll *et al.*, 1996). The purpose of applying a light force is to increase cellular activity without causing undue tissue compression and to prepare the tissues for further changes. Another reason is that it results in less discomfort and pain to the patient. Unmyelinated nerve endings persist in the hyalinised tissue, and are compressed during the initial stage.

The duration, equivalent to treatment time, is a more crucial factor than the magnitude of the force regarding adverse tissue reactions (Reitan 1964; Lindskog and Lilja, 1984; Owman-Moll *et al.*, 1996). Thus, a long

treatment period in an aging bone structure should be avoided.

The *direction* of forces will result in different kinds of tooth movements, often presented in terms of tipping, torque, bodily, intrusion, extrusion and rotation, resulting in different tissue response in the different parts of the PDL.

Orthodontic tooth movements

Tipping

Tipping of a tooth implies that a fulcrum is formed, resulting in a root movement in the opposite direction. The pressure is concentrated in limited areas of PDL, which results in formation of a hyalinised area below the alveolar crest as well as in the apical region (Figure 9.11). Tipping of a tooth by light continuous forces results in a greater movement within a shorter

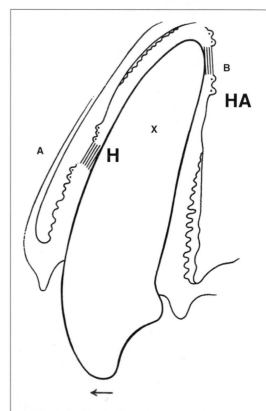

Figure 9.11 A tipping force of the tooth (the arrow show the force direction). Two hyalinised zones will be the result, one on the pressure side (H) and another in the apical region (HA). Centre of resistance (x).

time than that obtained by any other methods. In most young orthodontic patients, bone resorption resulting from a moderate tipping movement is usually followed by compensatory bone formation. The degree of such compensation varies individually and depends primarily of bone-forming osteoblasts in the periosteum (Reitan, 1967).

Torque

Torque is a tipping movement of the apex (Figure 9.12). During its initial phase, the pressure area is located in the middle part of the root. Later, the apical surface of the root gradually begins to compress adjacent periodontal fibres, establishing a wider pressure area. If more torque is incorporated into the arch-wire, the force will increase and may result in fenestration of the buccal bone plate (Figure 9.13).

Bodily movement

Bodily movement is obtained by establishing a couple of forces acting along parallel lines and distributing the force over the whole alveolar bone surface. This is a favourable method of displacement, provided that light continuous

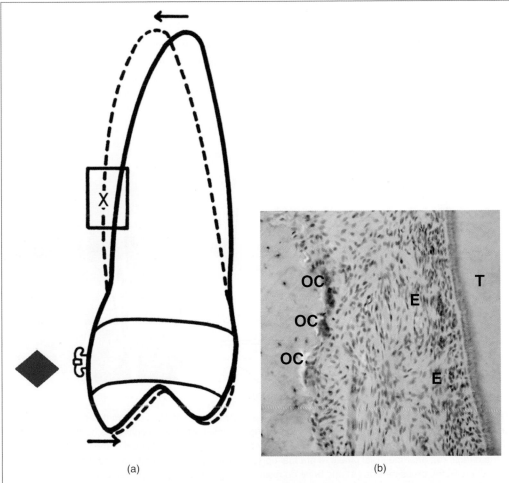

(a)   (b)

Figure 9.12 To the left (a), torqueing of a maxillary premolar. The arrows show the force directions and movements. The photomicrograph to the right (b), showing the pressure side in a 12-year-old patient after torqueing movement performed in the apical region with a force of 120cN during 2 weeks. As indicated by the presence of epithelial remnants, no hyalinization of the PDL has occurred. Tooth root surface (T), osteoclasts (OC) along the bone surface and epithelial remnants (E).

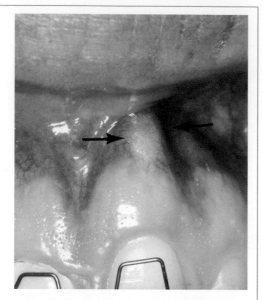

Figure 9.13 Torque movements resulting in bone fenestrations of the root tips of the left central and lateral incisors (arrows).

forces are applied to the tooth (Reitan, 1967). During its initial phase, a small compressed area of short duration is formed. No bodily movement is observed during this period; instead, a slight tipping occurs. The degree of this initial tipping varies according to the size of the arch and width of the brackets (Figure 9.14). The short duration of the hyalinisation results from an increased resorption on both sides of the hyalinised tissue on the pressure side, which leads to a rapid elimination of the hyalinised zone. This favourable reaction on the pressure side is caused by gradually increased stretching of fibre bundles on the tension side and the new bone layers along these fibres (Figure 9.14).

Rotation

Rotation of a tooth creates two pressure sides and two tension sides (Figure 9.15) and may cause certain variations in the type of tissue reaction on the pressure side (Reitan, 1967). Hyalinisation with undermining bone resorption,

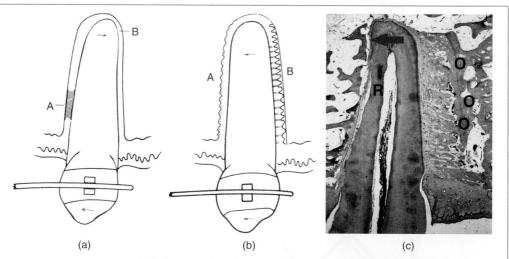

Figure 9.14 Two stages of bodily tooth movement; the arrows denote tooth movement directions. The drawing to the left (a), shows the effect observed during the initial stage of a continuous bodily movement. Hyalinised tissue/area (A) and slight compression (B), because of the initial tipping of the tooth. In the figure in the middle (b), after the initial phase, a gradual upright positioning of the tooth caused increased bone resorption on the pressure side (A) and bone deposition along the stretched fibre bundles (B). The photomicrograph to the right (c), shows a bodily movement, with the blue arrow showing the tooth movement direction of a premolar in a dog during a period of 6 months. New bone layers on the tension side with osteoblasts (O) and small root resorption on the pressure side (R).

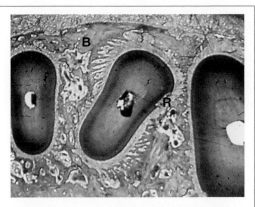

Figure 9.15 Experimental rotation of a maxillary second incisor in a dog. Formation of two pressure and tension sides. Demarcation line between old and new bone layers (B) and pressure side with root resorption (R).

and even root resorption, take place in one pressure zone, while direct bone resorption occurs on the other, variations caused by anatomy of the root and magnitude of the force. On the tension side, the bone spicules are formed along the stretched fibre bundles arranged obliquely. In the marginal region, rotation usually causes considerable displacement of fibrous structures. The free gingival fibre

groups are arranged obliquely from the root surface. Because they interface with the periosteal structures and the whole supra-alveolar fibre system, rotation also causes displacement of the fibrous tissue located some distance from the rotated tooth.

Extrusion

Extrusion ideally produces no areas of compression within the PDL, only tension. Varying with the individual tissue reaction, the periodontal fibre bundles elongate and new bone is deposited in areas of alveolar crest because of the tension exerted by these stretched fibres (Figure 9.16). In young individuals, extrusion of a tooth involves a more prolonged stretch and displacement of supra-alveolar fibre bundles than of the principle fibres in the middle and apical thirds of the PDL.

Intrusion

Unlike extruded teeth, intruded teeth in young individuals undergo minor positional changes. Stretch is exerted primarily on the principle fibres (Figure 9.16). Intrusion requires light force, because it is concentrated in a small area at the tooth apex with risk for apical root resorption.

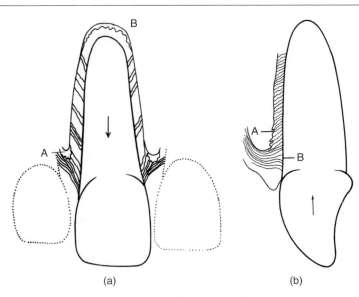

(a)   (b)

Figure 9.16 To the left (a), arrangement of fibre bundles during and after extrusion of a maxillary central incisor. New bone layers at the alveolar fundus (B). To the right (b), relaxation of the free gingival fibres during intrusion. Bone spicules laid down according to the direction of the fibre tension (A) and relaxed supra-alveolar tissue (B).

Conclusions

Application of an orthodontic force to a tooth results in a tooth movement, which depends on type, magnitude, direction and duration of the force. However, the transmission of the orthodontic force to a biological response in the periodontal tissues is not related to the mechanic sensing by the osteocytes as in the bone remodelling sequence. The accepted concept today is that an aseptic inflammation is the initiating factor for tooth movement. The tissue response in this process is of fundamental significance in making the proper use of biomechanical principles to avoid adverse tissue reactions.

REFERENCES

Brudvik, P. and Rygh, P. (1993) The initial phase of orthodontic root resorption incident to local compression of the periodontal ligament. Eur J Orthod 15: 249–263.

Brudvik, P. and Rygh, P. (1994) Multinucleated cells remove the main hyalinized tissue and start resorption of adjacent root surfaces. Eur J Orthod 16: 265–273.

Brudvik, P. and Rygh, P. (1995) Transition and determinants of orthodontic root resorption-repair sequence. Eur J Orthod 17: 177–188.

Davidovitch, Z., Nicolay, O.F., Ngan, P.W. *et al.* (1988) Neurotransmitters, cytokines, and the control of alveolar bone remodeling in orthodontics. Dent Clin North Am 32: 411–435.

Lindskog, S. and Lilja, E. (1984) Scanning electron microscopic study of orthodontically induced injuries to the periodontal membrane. Scand J Dent Res 92: 334–343.

Meikle, M.C. (2006) The tissue, cellular, and molecular regulation of orthodontic tooth movement: 100 years after Carl Sandstedt. Eur J Orthod 28: 221–240.

Owman-Moll, P., Kurol, J. and Lundgren, D. (1996) The effects of a four-fold increased orthodontic force magnitude on tooth movement and root resorption. An intra-individual study in adolescents. Eur J Orthod 18: 287–294.

Ransjö, M., Marklund, M., Persson, M. *et al.* (1998) Synergistic interactions of bradykinin, thrombin, interleukin 1 and tumor necrosis factor on prostanoid biosynthesis in human periodontal-ligament cells. Arch Oral Biol 43: 253–260.

Reitan, K. (1951) The initial tissue reaction incident to orthodontic tooth movement as related to the influence of function. An experimental histological study on animal and human material. Acta Odont Scand, Suppl 6: 1–240.

Reitan, K. (1964) Effects of force magnitude and direction of tooth movement on different alveolar types. Angle Orthod 34: 244–255.

Reitan, K. (1967) Clinical and histologic observations on tooth movement during and after orthodontic treatment. Am J Orthod 53: 721–745.

Rygh, P. (1972) Ultrastructural cellular reactions in pressure zones of rat molar periodontium incident to orthodontic tooth movement. Acta Odont Scand 30: 575–593.

Rygh, P. (1973) Ultrastructural changes of the periodontal fibres and their attachment in rat molar periodontium incident to orthodontic tooth movement. Scand J Dent Res 81: 467–480.

Sandstedt, C. (1904) Einige Beiträge zur Theorie der Zahnregulierung. Nord Tandl Tidsk 5: 236–256.

Wise, G.E. and King, G.J. (2008) Mechanisms of tooth eruption and tooth movement. J Dent Res 87: 414–434.

CHAPTER 10

Tissue response to orthopaedic forces

Birgit Thilander

Key topics

- Response in condyles
- Response in sutures

Learning objectives

- To understand the difference between orthopaedic and orthodontic forces
- To be able to describe the response in the TMJ region from functional appliances
- To understand the suture response to RME expansion
- To understand the TMJ response in a posterior functional crossbite

Essential Orthodontics, First Edition. Birgit Thilander, Krister Bjerklin and Lars Bondemark.
© 2018 John Wiley & Sons Ltd. Published 2018 by John Wiley & Sons Ltd.

Introduction

Orthopaedic forces are acting on the temporomandibular joint (TMJ region, when the position between the jaws is changed, and by that even the activity of the masticatory muscles, when the mandible is moved forward in Angle Class II cases by means of different types of orthodontic appliances (e.g. with an Andrésen activator or a Herbst appliance), or kept backwards in Angle Class III cases (e.g. with a chin-cap). Orthopaedic forces are also acting on the maxillary sutures by moving the maxilla into a forward position or a restraint of forward growth of the maxilla (e.g. by means of a facemask or a headgear), or in expanding the intra-maxillary suture (e.g. with rapid maxillary expansion (RME)) in patients with crossbite. Thus, orthopaedic forces differ from orthodontic forces, which are acting on the teeth and their adjacent structures, resulting in tooth movements within the jaws.

Whether functional appliances or orthopaedic forces can enhance or diminish the condylar and sutural growth is an academic issue, and therefore will be discussed in this chapter.

Response in condyles

The major aim of dentofacial orthodontic treatment in Class II individuals with mandibular retrognathia is to enhance or optimize the growth of the condyle by functional anterior displacement of the mandible, while in Class III subjects, the treatment aims to restrain the mandibular growth. The extent to which this can be achieved, and whether it has any clinical significance, are topics of long-standing controversy. Both rat and monkey models have been used to study condylar adaptation to protrusive forces, while its adaptation to retrusive forces has been of minor interest. The response in the condylar cartilage to orthopaedic forces has been of special interest in most experimental studies.

Experimental studies

Experimental studies on rats with anterior displacement of the mandible have demonstrated an increase in the thickness of the proliferating zone (PZ) with an increased number of dividing cells, while mandibular retrusion with chin-cap therapy revealed a reduced thickness of PZ and a decreased number of cells (Petrovic, 1972). In follow-up studies in the rat, Petrovic *et al.* (1975) reported that anterior displacement of the mandible in the growing rat results in additional growth of the condylar cartilage, by stimulating the cells of the PZ to undergo mitosis. However, subsequent experiments in rats, using biochemical, histomorphometric and autoradiographic methods, have not been able to support this statement. Furthermore, experiments in changing the design of the appliance, for example the degree of opening, forward displacement of the mandible, have also been presented (Ghafari and Degroote, 1986; Tsolakis and Spyropoulos, 1997). Although linear measurements indicated an increase of the mandibular length, it was impossible to explain that this was due to an increase in the growth of the condylar cartilage.

While the evidence from rat experiments has been controversial, anterior displacement of the mandible in the rhesus monkey has shown significant morphological changes in the TMJ region. The first to provide convincing histological evidence that anterior displacement of the mandible caused remodelling of the glenoid fossa and condyle was Carl Breitner (1940). Some subsequent studies have verified his original findings and shown that the TMJ in monkeys is capable of functional adaptation (Baume and Derechsweiler, 1961; Stöckli and Willert, 1971). The anterior displacement of the mandible changed the normal dental relationship into a Class III malocclusion, involving a change even in the facial muscles (McNamara, 1973), especially an increased activity of the lateral pterygoid muscles. A modification of the neuromuscular pattern was also observed with a skeleton adaptation to the experimental conditions. Histologically, changes in cartilaginous growth were observed in the condyle, particularly along its posterior border, and even in the articular fossa. However, after about 10 weeks, the remodelling process was completed.

Changes in the condylar cartilage occur during a short period of treatment and thus seem to be of secondary importance in response to orthopaedic forces. Studies in which mandibular condyles were transplanted into a nonfunctional environment have shown that the progenitor cells of the PZ differentiate into osteoblasts, and not into chondroblasts as *in situ* (Duterloo, 1967). The cells are therefore multipotential and can form either cartilage or bone, depending upon the environmental circumstances. Finally, the articular zone of the cartilage is a continuation of the fibrous and cellular layers of the periosteum, and hence can adapt to alterations in the mechanical equilibrium of the skeleton. Thus, a forward displacement of the mandible is followed by adaptive changes in the TMJ-region with altered growth direction (Meikle, 2007).

Clinical application

Mandibular protrusion in Angle Class II cases, resulting in remodelling of the TMJ, in monkeys is one thing and remodelling in the clinic is quite another, even if the condyle of the monkey undergoes an age-dependent change in growth direction, which might be an indicator for treatment of growing children with functional appliances (Luder, 1987). However, the clinician is aiming at changing an abnormal growth pattern into a more normal one, just the opposite of what is done in animal experiments, i.e. to shift the jaw from a normal into an abnormal position. In addition, a controlled environment concerning cooperation comparable to that in animal studies is hardly attainable in patients. Furthermore, cephalometric measurements suffer from identification of some landmarks (e.g. condylon), and from errors of projection. Linear measurements are often given in millimetres, without paying attention to the magnification factor, which usually varies between 5 and 14%. It should also be noted that the distance between condylon and pogonion, calculated from landmarks in the mid-sagittal plane, is different from its real distance in the lateral view. Those factors must be considered when describing the orthopaedic effect of an appliance. The individual growth potential during the treatment period is also included in this effect. It is, however, impossible to distinguish the effect of the appliance from the normal growth of the patient during the treatment period and it is difficult or impossible to give an exact value of the effect of the different functional appliances.

Mandibular retrusion in Angle Class III cases has focused clinically on different appliances, for example Frankel regulator III or chin-cap, often in combination with a facemask. Some cephalometric studies have shown that chin-cap treatment in the young individual may improve the Class III occlusion through a retropositioning of the mandible (Thilander, 1995; Allen *et al.,* 1993; Deguchi *et al.,* 2002), due to remodelling in the TMJ-region and not due to a retardation of the mandibular growth.

The response to orthopaedic forces is not only of interest from sagittal aspects as described in cephalometry (e.g. Angle Classes II and III), but also in transversal dimension. A forced guidance of the mandible will result in asymmetric activity of the masticatory muscles, significantly lower on the non-crossbite side (Troelstrup and Möller, 1970; Ingervall and Thilander, 1975; Ferrario *et al.,* 1999). The adaptive changes of the jaw muscles vary with intensity and duration of the stimuli. In general, stretch increases the neuromuscular activity while pressure reduces the neuromuscular activity and hence may change the fibre-type composition. Of importance was the finding that the asymmetric muscle activity was documented not only in the inter-maxillary position but also in the rest position (Ingervall and Thilander, 1975), which suggests that the relaxed mandible was still displaced to the crossbite side (Figure 10.1) due to a neuromuscular adaptation to the intercuspal relationship (ICP).

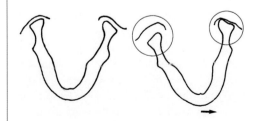

Figure 10.1 To the left, normal occlusion with bilateral normal position of the mandible condyle in the fossae. To the right, a unilateral left posterior crossbite has resulted in changed condylar position in the glenoid fossae.

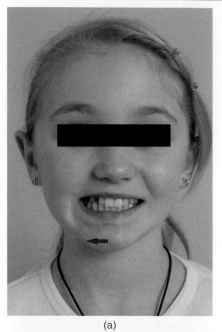

(a)

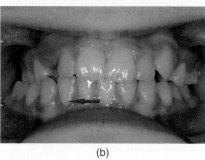

(b)

Figure 10.2 In (a), deviation of the chin to the posterior crossbite side (red arrow), resulting in a facial asymmetry of the young girl. In (b), the unilateral crossbite (red arrow indicates deviation to the right side). In (c), a young adult with an untreated unilateral right-sided posterior crossbite. Deviation of the chin to the right (red arrow).

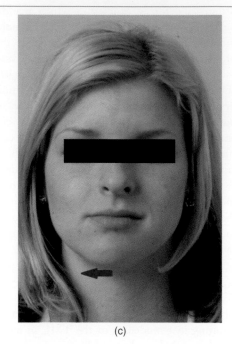

(c)

Figure 10.2 (*Continued*)

early treatment from growth-adaptive as well as from neuromuscular reason is indicated. Left untreated, there is a great risk that the functional crossbite in young ages will be transformed into a cranial skeletal asymmetry and malocclusion in later ages (Figure 10.2) (Thilander and Bjerklin, 2012).

Response in sutures

Facial sutures provide a firm union between adjacent bones. However, in response to mechanical forces, they permit slight movements of the bony parts. The structure of the tissue, especially its fibrous component, varies with age as well as within the same suture, as described in Chapter 3. Changes in the positional relationships of the bones of the facial skeleton in the posterior, anterior and transversal directions have been demonstrated in animals with different techniques.

Experimental studies

In monkeys, forces have been applied to move the maxilla in a forward or backward position

In addition, when the mandible is displaced into ICP, the condyle on the non-crossbite side will move in a downward-medial direction and the condyle on the crossbite side in an upward-lateral direction, resulting in a changed condylar position in the glenoid fossae. Moreover, such a changed condylar/temporal relationship will have an influence on the remodelling processes in those areas (Thilander 1995; Hesse *et al.,* 1997; Nerder *et al.,* 1999; Pinto *et al.,* 2001; Kecik *et al.,* 2007). Thus,

by means of headgear. It has been shown that, during the late deciduous dentition stage, the midfacial complex can be moved posteriorly into a Class III relationship within a few months by using heavy continuous extra-oral forces (Bousseau and Kubisch, 1977). However, this effect is transitional as the maxilla resumed its forward growth pattern after termination of the high-pull traction (Tuenge and Elder, 1974). Extra-oral forward traction to move the maxilla to an anterior position with heavy forces in young monkeys has also shown displacement of the maxillary complex after a few months (Kanbara, 1977), but during the post-treatment period a general reversal of these changes was observed after removal of the headgear.

Histological studies have confirmed that the displacement seen cephalometrically is mediated by resorption and remodelling of the facial sutures (Droschl, 1975). The serpentine configuration with inter-digitations disappears, the fibres lose their orientation, and active osteoclasts are seen on the bone surfaces. This stage of direct resorption is frequently preceded by local hyalinisation (Linge, 1973). Heavy extra-oral forces have shown sutural opening associated with fewer inter-digitations in the circum-maxillary sutures. Reorganisation and formation of new inter-digitations will occur when the orthopaedic force is removed. Thus, the suture will react to pressure much in the same way as seen on the alveolar bone surface of the PDL in tooth movements.

Clinical application

While numerous studies in monkeys have shown that mechanical forces of appropriate strength and duration can remodel facial sutures, the extent to which these changes can be utilized clinically continues to be the subject of debate. However, according to experimental studies, we can conclude that it is possible to influence the sutures, especially in early developmental periods, with use of skeletal anchorage. The degree and direction of the orthopaedic force (cervical versus occipital) will also influence the outcome of the forward and backward distraction, depending upon whether the sutures are exposed to a tensile or a compressive mechanical strain.

Maxillary protraction

For maxillary protraction in treatment of Class III malocclusion, the orthopaedic facemask can be used (Delaire *et al.*, 1978). However, the degree to which the maxillary distraction can be achieved clinically is age and technique dependent. The drawback of applying forces directly to the teeth is their tendency to move, thereby reducing the orthopaedic effect. Skeletal anchorage, introduced by Turley *et al.* (1980), has therefore been used to exert the force directly on the bone via endosseous implants. Skeletal anchorage by mini-screws (TADs) nowadays is a matter of course, as they will provide forward distraction directly to the bones and hence minimise unwanted tooth movements.

Transversal displacement

Widening of the median palatine suture, often by RME, has been an accepted clinical procedure for many years. The method, first presented by Angell (1860), was met with scepticism, until Haas (1965) showed that a fixed palatal expander in adolescents had a favourable influence on the outcome, and today is a clinically well-documented procedure in orthodontics. This treatment is an example of osteogenetic distraction, which means that not only the mid-palatal suture, but also the circum-maxillary sutures, have to be remodelled. Thus, a complex suture system is involved in the term 'maxillary expansion', and consequently the often-used 'rapid palatal expansion' is an incorrect term.

Maxillary expansion

Maxillary expansion, aimed at widening the inter-maxillary suture, needs a stationary anchorage, and the optimal treatment period is during the mixed dentition with no or few bone bridges in the suture (Figure 10.3). The mechanical response to traction includes changes in the orientation of the fibre bundles. A positive correlation exists between the magnitude of the tensile force and osteogenic response. Osteoblasts and Sharpey's fibres are incorporated into the bone surfaces by the deposition of new bone layers, while the suture will react to tension in the same way as seen on the alveolar bone surface of the PDL. When the

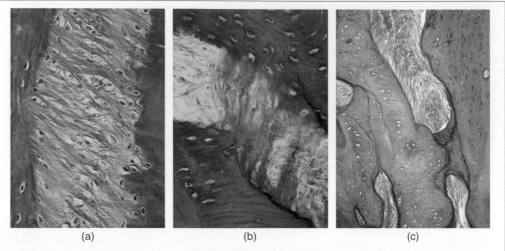

Figure 10.3 Photomicrographs from the human intermaxillary suture. To the left (a), in young ages the collagen fibres perpendicular to the bony surface. In the middle (b), the thickness and density of fibres have increased with age. To the right (c), after 14 years of age, a stage to bony obliteration.

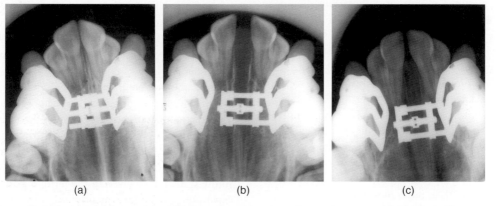

Figure 10.4 To the left (a), a rapid maxillary appliance has been inserted to expand the intermaxillary suture, no expansion yet started. In the middle (b), after 21 days of expansion and a clearly widened suture. To the right (c), deposition of bone in the widened suture to allow the suture to recover.

orthopaedic force is removed, reorganisation with normalisation of the width and the formation of new inter-digitation will occur. The deposition of bone that accompanies traction allows the suture to recover (Figure 10.4).

When the suture is ossified and 'closed', surgical intervention should be done. In the literature, the terms 'slow' and 'rapid' expansion are often used to explain differences in the outcome of the treatment.

Conclusions

Whether functional appliances or orthopaedic forces can stimulate or diminish the condylar growth is still an academic issue. However, it can be stated that mandibular displacement through orthopaedic appliances initiates remodelling activity within the TMJ and alters the condylar growth direction, particularly in an actively growing individual.

It is possible to influence the facial sutures, especially in early developmental periods with use of skeletal anchorage. The degree and direction of the orthopaedic force will influence the outcome of the forward, backward or transversal distraction, depending upon whether the sutures are exposed to a tensile or a compressive mechanical strain.

The facial sutures will react to pressure and tension much in the same way as seen on the alveolar bone surface of the PDL in tooth movements.

REFERENCES

Allen, R., Connolly, I. and Richardson, A. (1993) Early treatment of Class III incisor relationship using the chincap appliance. Eur J Orthod 15: 371–376.

Angell, E. (1860) Treatment of irregularity of the permanent or adult teeth. Dent Cos 1: 540–544.

Baume, L. and Derechsweiler, H. (1961) Is the condylar growth centre responsive to orthodontic therapy? An experimental study in *Macaca mulatta*. J Oral Surg Oral Med Oral Pathol 14: 347–362.

Bousseau, M. and Kubisch, R. (1977) Continuous versus intermittent extra oral traction. An experimental study. Am J Orthod 71: 607–621.

Breitner, C. (1940) Bone changes resulting from experimental orthodontic treatment. Am J Orthod 26: 521–547.

Deguchi, T., Kuroda, T., Minoshima, Y. *et al.* (2002) Craniofacial features of patients with Class III abnormalities: growth-related changes and effects of long-term chincup therapy. Am J Orthod Dentofacial Orthop 121: 84–92.

Delaire, J, Verdon, P. and Flour, J. (1978) Möglichkeiten und Grenzen extraoraler Kräfte in postero-anteriorer Richtung unter Verwendung der orthopädischen Maske. Fort Kieferortop 38: 27–45.

Droschl, H. (1975) The effect of heavy orthopaedic forces on suture of the facial bones. Angle Orthod 45: 26–33.

Duterloo, H. (1967) *In vivo* implantation of the mandible condyle of the rat. An experimental investigation of the growth of the lower jaw. University of Nijmegen, The Netherlands. (Thesis)

Ferrario, V., Sforza, C. and Serrao, G. (1999) The influence of crossbite on the coordinated electromyographic activity of human masticatory muscles during mastication. J Oral Rehab 26: 575–581.

Ghafari, J. and Degroote, C. (1986) Condylar cartilage response to continuous mandibular displacement in the rat. Angle Orthod 56: 49–57.

Haas, A. (1965) The treatment of maxillary deficiency by opening the midpalatal suture. Angle Orthod 35: 200–217.

Hesse, K., Artun, J., Joondeph, D. *et al.* (1997) Changes in condylar position and occlusion associated with maxillary expansion for correction of functional unilateral posterior crossbite. Am J Orthod Dentofacial Orthop 111: 410–418.

Ingervall, B. and Thilander, B. (1975) Activity of temporal and masseter muscles in children with a lateral forced bite. Angle Orthod 45: 249–258.

Kanbara, T. (1977) Dentofacial changes produced by extraoral forward force in the *Macaca irus*. Am J Orthod 71: 249–277.

Kecik, D., Kocadereli, I. and Saatci, I. (2007) Evaluation of the treatment changes of functional posterior crossbite in the mixed dentition. Am J Orthod Dentofacial Orthop 131: 202–215.

Linge, L. (1973) Tissue changes in facial sutures incident to mechanical influences. An experimental study in *Macaca mulatta*. University of Oslo, Norway. (Thesis)

Luder, H. (1987) Growth direction in the mandibular condyle of prepubertal and pubertal monkeys (*Macaca fascicularis*) studied by morphometry and radioautography. Arch Oral Biol 32: 239–247.

McNamara, J.A. (1973) Neuromuscular and skeletal adaptations to altered function in the orofacial region. Am J Orthod 64: 578–606.

Meikle, M.C. (2007) Remodeling the dentofacial skeleton: the biological basis of orthodontics and dentofacial orthopedics. J Dent Res 86: 12–24.

Nerder, P., Bakke, M. and Solow, B. (1999) The functional shift of the mandible in unilateral posterior crossbite and the adaptation of the temporomandibular joint: a pilot study. Eur J Orthod 21: 155–166.

Petrovic, A. (1972) Mechanisms and regulation of mandibular condylar growth. Acta Morphol Neerl Scand 10: 25–34.

Petrovic, A., Stutzmann, J. and Oudet, C. (1975) Control processes in the postnatal growth of the condylar cartilage of the mandible. In: *Craniofacial Growth Series, Centre for Human Growth and Development*. Ann Arbor, University of Michigan, pp. 101–153.

Pinto, A., Buschang, P., Throckmorton, G. *et al.* (2001) Morphological and positional asymmetries of young children with functional unilateral posterior crossbite. Am J Orthod Dentofacial Orthop 120: 513–520.

Stöckli, P. and Willert, H. (1971) Tissue reactions in the temporomandibular joint resulting from anterior displacement of the mandible in the monkey. Am J Orthod 60: 142–155.

Thilander, B. (1995) Basic mechanisms in craniofacial growth. Acta Odont Scand 53: 144–151.

Thilander, B. and Bjerklin, K. (2012) Posterior crossbite and temporomandibular disorders (TMDs): need for orthodontic treatment? Eur J Orthod 34: 667–673.

Troelstrup, B. and Möller, E. (1970) Electromyography of the temporalis and masseter muscles in children with unilateral forced posterior cross-bite. Scand J Dent Res 78: 425–430.

Tsolakis, A. and Spyropoulos, M. (1997) An appliance designed for experimental mandibular hyperpropulsion in rats. Eur J Orthod 19: 1–7.

Tuenge, R. and Elder, J. (1974) Post-treatment changes following extraoral high-pull traction to the maxilla of *Macaca mulatta*. Am J Orthod Oral Surg 66: 618–644.

Turley, P., Shapiro, P. and Moffett, B. (1980) The loading of bio-glass-coated aluminium oxide implants to produce sutural expansion of the maxillary complex in the pigtail monkey (*Macaca nemestrina*). Arch Oral Biol 25: 459–469.

CHAPTER 11
Possible adverse tissue reactions

Birgit Thilander and Lars Bondemark

Key topics

- White spot lesion
- Root resorption
- Gingivitis and loss of marginal bone support
- Bone dehiscence
- Allergic reactions
- Pain and injuries of appliance
- Risk of temporomandibular disorder (TMD)

Learning objectives

- To understand how to avoid white spot lesions
- To be able to describe risk factors in apical root resorption
- To understand and describe orthodontic tooth movements in labial/buccal direction as a risk factor to bone dehiscence
- To understand problems with orthodontics in Nickel-sensitive individuals
- To describe possible risk-factors for TMD in orthodontic patients

Essential Orthodontics, First Edition. Birgit Thilander, Krister Bjerklin and Lars Bondemark.
© 2018 John Wiley & Sons Ltd. Published 2018 by John Wiley & Sons Ltd.

Introduction

Many studies have, despite insufficient scientific evidence, emphasised the need for orthodontic treatment due to unfavourable consequences of several malocclusions such as crowding (predisposition to gingivitis), functional crossbites (risk of developing of temporomandibular dysfunction), open bite (deficient chewing capacity), proclined maxillary incisors (risk of traumatic injuries), and impacted teeth (risk of root resorption). On the other hand, an orthodontic treatment may in some cases initiate some adverse effects, and clinical studies have from time to time reported that orthodontic treatment may cause damage to the teeth and their supporting tissues. This chapter aims to point out some possible adverse tissue reactions to avoid complications in the orthodontic clinic.

Damage to teeth

White spot lesions

It is generally regarded that treatment with fixed orthodontic appliances can cause enamel demineralization adjacent to the brackets, because of accumulation of aciduric and acidogenic bacteria (Chapman et al., 2010). This enamel demineralization, called white spot lesions (WSL), is an unwanted clinical problem with a reported prevalence of 15 to 85% (Chapman et al., 2010; Sonesson et al., 2014). The WSL have limited ability to improve after fixed appliance removal and therefore the final esthetical result may be jeopardized (Figure 11.1). There

exists various strategies to prevent WSL during treatment and evidence is found that fluoride varnishes, gels and high-fluoride tooth paste or fluoride-containing bonding materials could be fluoride supplement alternatives to reduce the incidence and severity of WSL adjacent to bracket and bands (Derks et al., 2004; Sonesson et al., 2014).

Since food debris and plaque are risk factors for WSL and gingivitis, it is very important to apply a suitable hygiene programme with topical fluoride administration for every individual patient. To learn from this is: Do not start an orthodontic treatment until the patient can understand and practise plaque control.

Pulpal reaction

When removing the bond material left at the enamel surfaces after debonding, there is a risk that increased temperature will result in pulp damage (Vukovich et al., 1991). Thus, the use of water-cooling is especially important in this procedure. Orthodontic extrusion and intrusion have been associated with vascular changes and pulpal oedema in adult patients. Those rare disturbances seem to be more severe when greater forces are applied for a longer time.

Root resorption

Root resorption continuous to be one of the most frequent lesion, associated with orthodontic treatment (Kurol et al., 1996; Weltman et al., 2010; Lund et al., 2012). There are two types of root resorption: one appears as small superficial

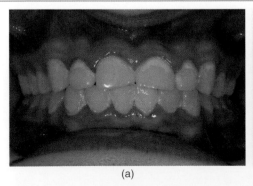
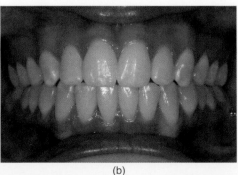

(a)   (b)

Figure 11.1 In (a), general WSLs after 1.5 years of treatment with fixed appliance, and in (b), another patient showing normal enamel conditions after fixed appliance therapy.

resorptions, associated with the hyaline zone, and undergoes repair, while the other is localised at the apex of the root and leads to shortening of the root.

Resorption at tooth surface

By electron microscopy, Kvam (1972) demonstrated resorption defects in the periphery of the hyalinised zone (Figure 11.2). A side effect of the cellular activity during removal of the necrotic hyalinised tissue is that the cementoid layer of the root is left with a raw unprotected surface, which is attacked by resorptive cells that resemble the osteoclast in structural and functional aspects (Brudvik and Rygh, 1994). Root resorption then occurs around this cell-free tissue, starting at the border of the hyalinised zone. The first sign of root resorption (initial phase) is a penetration of cells from the periphery of the necrotic tissue where mononucleated fibroblast-like cells, stained negatively by tartrate-resistant acid and phosphatase (TRAP), start to attack the precementum/cementum surface. Root resorption beneath the main hyalinised zone occurs in a later phase, during which multinucleated TRAP-positive cells are involved in removing the main mass of necrotic PDL tissue and in resorbing the outer layer of the root cementum, opposite to the TRAP-negative cells that are involved, even in the resorption of the bone surface. Those results support the statement by Tanaka *et al.* (1990), where separate clast cells are resorbing bone and tooth structures simultaneously.

When the orthodontic force has terminated, repair starts with a synthesis of collagen fibres by fibroblast/cementoblast-like cells, and new cementum is deposited on the root surface simultaneously with re-establishment of the new PDL. However, resorption continues in the area where hyalinised tissue persists, even after active force had terminated (Brudvik and Rygh, 1995). For the clinician, it is important to know that minor resorption lacunae can be repaired during periods of no force or possibly during periods of extremely low force application.

Resorption at tooth apex

Apical root resorption (Figure 11.3) is a multifactorial problem and a serious complication in orthodontic treatment. It is known that root resorption is the result of cell activity, and the osteoclast is the inevitable cell during tooth movement, but the biological factors triggering the process are not yet fully understood. However, the decisive factors for developing root resorption appear to be controlled primarily by the pulp status and the extent of injury to the innermost cells in the periodontal ligament (PDL). Teeth in a formative stage display less root resorption during orthodontic tooth movement.

Ketcham (1929) was first to report on apical root resorption in vital permanent teeth, and he found that the maxillary incisors are more frequently involved than other teeth, a statement verified by many later clinical studies. Tendency to resorption is greater in teeth with invagination and pipette-shaped roots (Levander and Malmgren, 1988) and in dentitions with agenesis (Kjaer, 1995). Trauma to maxillary incisors before orthodontic treatment is a factor strongly associated with resorption during treatment.

Most findings indicate that orthodontic forces in terms of magnitude, direction and duration are important for an understanding of the resorptive process; the duration of the force is more critical than the magnitude.

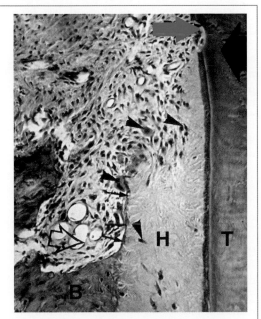

Figure 11.2 The green arrow pointing to a superficial resorption defect of the root and the defect rather close to the hyalinised zone (H). The alveolar bone (B) and root surface of the tooth (T).

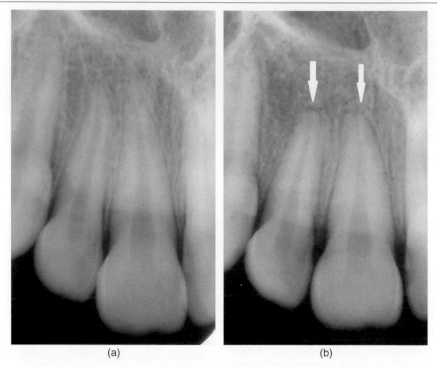

(a) (b)

Figure 11.3 In (a), maxillary right central and lateral incisor before orthodontic treatment, and in (b), the same teeth after treatment and with minor (2–3 mm) apical root resorptions (white arrows).

Furthermore, correction of overjet and intrusion of teeth are significantly correlated to apical root resorption. The type of the orthodontic appliance thus appears to be of importance.

Although the cause and mechanism remain unknown, it is known that there are *high-risk* teeth and certain types of patients who are particularly susceptible. The degree of root resorption is usually less than 2 mm, but can be more extensive in some cases.

Although radiographs do not disclose root resorption at an early stage of the orthodontic treatment, *X-ray inspection* of orthodontic patients is recommended. The first inspection should take place during the treatment, as root resorption proceeds very rapidly in some patients, and continued controls thus are of importance.

Damage to tooth-supporting tissues

Gingival inflammation caused by bacterial plaque at the gingival margin (Figure 11.4) is characterised by great plaque index, bleeding tendency and pocket depth, and has been observed more frequently in molars with orthodontic bands than in bonded ones (Boyd and Baumrind, 1992). A highly probably explanation for these differences is the difficulty in plaque removal on the gingival margin of the bands. An alternative explanation for at least part of the attachment loss is the mechanical injury caused by the placement of the bands too deep into the gingival pocket.

Gingival recession, i.e. displacement of the soft tissue margin apical to the cement-enamel junction (CEJ) with exposure of the root surface can be observed in combination with orthodontic treatment, especially with alignment and proclination of crowded incisors (Figure 11.5). An experimental study in the monkey could demonstrate that the apical displacement of the gingival margin was a result of a reduced soft tissue thickness of the free gingiva (Wennström *et al.*, 1987). The volume of the covering soft tissue should be considered as a factor that may develop gingival retraction during or after active orthodontic treatment. Thus, the tooth should

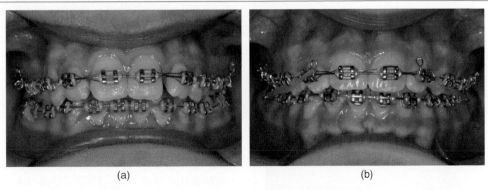

Figure 11.4 In (a), a patient with fixed appliance showing general gingival inflammation and bad oral hygiene. In (b), another patient showing how the oral hygiene should appear when treatment with fixed appliance is performed.

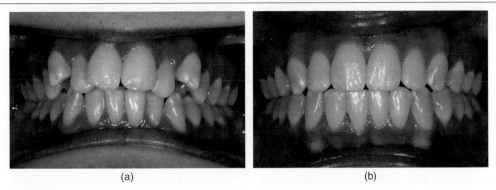

Figure 11.5 In (a), before treatment of crowding, and in (b), the same patient after treatment (proclination of mandibular incisors) and a small gingival recession has occurred (blue arrow).

be moved within the envelope of the alveolar process by a light force, and with bone, not through bone.

Labial and buccal tooth movements will displace the roots towards, and accidentally through, the thin cortical plate, i.e. bone dehiscence. So for example, a torqueing movement may displace the apex of the root through the cortical bone, resulting in fenestration (Figure 11.6). Contrary to a bone fenestration, localised to the apical part of the root, a bone dehiscence involves marginal bone loss at the labial/buccal aspect of the root. An experimental study in the Beagle dog demonstrated that bone dehiscence can be produced in the buccal alveolar bone by moving incisors in a labial direction, not accompanied by loss of connective attachment. A retention period of 5 months in this displaced tooth position

could not demonstrate any sign of bone formation of the dehiscence, presumably due to a degradation of both the organic and inorganic components of the bone, including osteogenic cells because of the orthodontic force. When the teeth were moved back to their original position, a complete regeneration of the alveolar bone took place. The mechanism of this reversal of bone loss is not known, but it seems logical to assume that cells with the capacity to form bone may have invaded the area of bone dehiscence on the labial aspect of the teeth during their movement back to their original position.

Clinical studies have demonstrated that orthodontically treated patients showed larger mean values for the distance between the CEJ and the alveolar crest compared to controls (non-treated subjects). The observed differences were small, between 0.1 and 0.5 mm

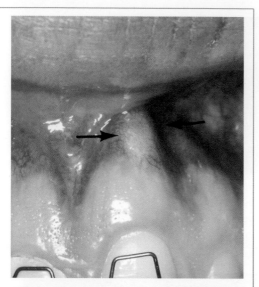

Figure 11.6 The apex of the maxillary left central incisor has been displaced through the cortical bone (arrows), because of too much torqueing movement.

of tooth morphology leading to plaque accumulation. Even if the majority of the patients presented little or no damage, it must be pointed out that a small number of patients showed considerably more damage, especially those who had difficulties with the oral hygiene regimen during treatment. This observation indicates that orthodontic treatment can aggravate a pre-existing plaque-induced gingival lesion, causing loss of alveolar bone and periodontal attachment, resulting in infra-bony pockets (Ericsson *et al.*, 1977). These findings indeed deserve attention in patients who have been treated for periodontal disease, especially at intruding and tilting movements. Thus, gingival pockets have to be eliminated before starting the orthodontic treatment.

Allergic reactions

There has been particular interest in the extent and cause of skin lesions in orthodontic patients, as well as in orthodontic staff members. Skin lesions on the hands of the staff were related to exposure to dental materials, especially etching/bonding agents, and the use of gloves (Altuna *et al.*, 1991), later verified by others.

It has been reported that 0.4% of patients show allergic reactions during orthodontic treatment and the reactions are often caused by contact between the skin and the extra oral face bow in the headgear (Jacobsen and Hensten-Pettersen, 2003). The allergic reactions consist in most cases of nickel allergy, manifested

(Figure 11.7), and regarded as clinically irrelevant (Hollender *et al.*, 1980; Aass and Gjermo, 1992; Bondemark, 1998). However, it should not go unrecognized that loss of alveolar bone support also occurs as a normal function of aging under normal conditions (Albander *et al.*, 1986).

The small changes in marginal bone support for orthodontic patients are considered to be a direct consequence of either band placement, tipping or extrusive effects or because

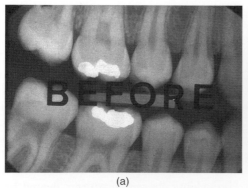
(a)

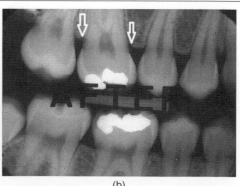
(b)

Figure 11.7 In (a), bitewing radiograph showing the marginal bone level before orthodontic treatment. In (b), after 2 years of treatment with a fixed appliance using bands on first molars. The white arrows indicate a loss of marginal bone of approximately 0.1 to 0.3 mm on the mesial and distal surface of the maxillary right molar.

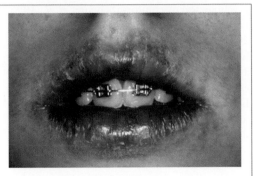

Figure 11.8 Pronounced oedema and erythema of the lips in a nickel-sensitive patient treated with fixed appliance of stainless steel.

as an itchy, blistering, erythematous rash on, for example, the cheeks and lips (Figure 11.8). Nickel allergy is a type 4 cell mediated response, i.e. 24 to 48 hours after exposure to the allergen, the reaction is clinically noticeable. It has been described that the prevalence of nickel allergy in different populations is 8 to 19%, and girls or women predominate over men, ratio 1:5 (Feasby *et al.*, 1988; Kerosuo *et al.*, 1996; Fors *et al.*, 2012). Furthermore, body piercing is strongly correlated to nickel hypersensitivity, which means that the prevalence is increased up to 30% after piercing (Kerosuo *et al.*, 1996).

Even if orthodontic treatment with fixed appliances contain nickel, the release of nickel ions from a bimaxillary fixed appliance is approximately 10 µg, and this release corresponds to 3 to 10% of the daily food intake of nickel (Flyvholm *et al.*, 1984). It has also been demonstrated that the nickel content of saliva can increase directly after the insertion of orthodontic appliances, but after a while (weeks to months , nickel ions are not be detected.

Overall, there exists no indication that orthodontic treatment with nickel containing appliances increases the prevalence of nickel hypersensitivity. The explanation may be that it requires a 12-fold higher concentration of nickel in the oral mucosa in comparison with the skin to obtain an intra oral reaction, since the antigen presenting cells (Langerhans cells) are much fewer in the epithelium of the oral mucosa compared to the epithelium in the skin. Furthermore, the glycoproteins in the saliva protect and the saliva 'washes away' the nickel ions.

From different animal studies it have been reported that increased nickel intake through food, as well as oral exposure of nickel from orthodontic appliances, induce a tolerance to later develop a nickel sensitivity. Anyhow, before starting an orthodontic treatment in a nickel-sensitive patient, it is recommended to use plastic encased outer bows of a headgear, brackets made of titanium or ceramics, nickel-free arch wires (e.g. titanium molybden arch wire), and avoid soldering since it increases the nickel ion release (Figure 11.9).

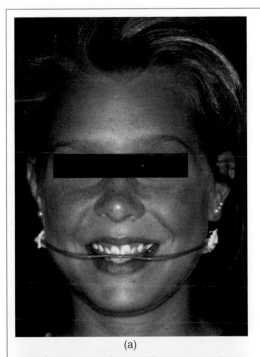

(a)

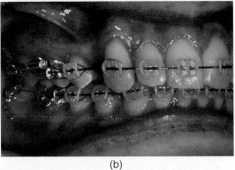

(b)

Figure 11.9 In (a), a nickel-sensitive patient using a plastic encased outer bow of a headgear. In (b), another nickel-sensitive patient bonded with brackets made of ceramics and in whom bands of titanium and a titanium molybdenum arch wire have been inserted.

In a patient who is not allergic to nickel, the risk is virtually non-existent to develop a nickel allergy because of the nickel-containing appliance. If some form of piercing is planned and orthodontic treatment is discussed, it is appropriate to carry out the orthodontic treatment first, since a slow and low concentration release of nickel ions from the orthodontic appliance means a tolerance of a developing nickel allergy in the future (Kerosuo et al., 1996; Fors et al., 2012).

Pain during orthodontic treatment

Pain has been reported to be the patients' major concern during orthodontic treatment and studies on adolescents and adults show that 95% of patients report pain experiences during treatment (Bergius et al., 2000; Scheurer et al., 1996). It can also be noted that pain experiences are subjective and multidimensional and comprise sensory as well as affective aspects. The degree of pain cannot only be explained by the force of application or different types of appliances, but also by several factors such as emotional, cognitive, environmental and cultural factors.

Pain and discomfort are mainly reported during the first week after insertion of an orthodontic appliance. Pain scores an overall peak between 12 hours and 3 days after insertion and the scores return to baseline at day 7 (Johal et al., 2014; Wiedel and Bondemark, 2016), and remain at baseline level throughout the whole treatment period (Feldmann et al., 2012).

It is not clear whether gender differences exist, but it has been shown that girls experience more pain and more often use analgesics than boys do during orthodontic treatment (Scheurer et al., 1996; Feldmann et al., 2012).

Overall, the general pain and discomfort levels often are low to moderate, but there exist few patients who really suffer severely from pain during orthodontic treatment. Consequently, medication for relief of pain is common during the first week of treatment (Scheurer et al., 1996; Feldmann et al., 2012). In addition, pain associated with orthodontic treatment has a potential impact on daily life, primarily as psychological discomfort (Scheurer et al., 1996; Feldmann et al., 2012; Wiedel and Bondemark, 2016). Moreover, swallowing, speech and jaw function can be altered during treatment, as well as difficulties in chewing hard food (Feldmann et al., 2012; Wiedel and Bondemark, 2016). It is advisable to give thorough information to patients about pain, and pain management should be a routine measure before and during orthodontic treatment.

Risk of temporomandibular disorders (TMD)

It has been postulated that orthodontic treatment may change the function of the stomatognathic system and thus be a potential risk for TMD. In spite of the abundant bibliography on this subject, conflicting opinions still exist. Differences as regards selection of subjects (age and number) and methods (examination or questionnaire) may be one explanation. Another reason is that most studies are cross-sectional or retrospective. Longitudinal studies, however, support the conclusion that orthodontic therapy in children and adolescents, from a general point of view, is not a risk for the development of TMD (Sadowsky and Polsen, 1984; Dibbets and van der Weele, 1987; Egermark and Thilander, 1992; Henrikson, 1999).

TMD is a generic term for a number of clinical signs and symptoms involving the TMJs and masticatory muscles. An uncertain relationship between signs and symptoms has been questioned as the patient's complaints might be seen as unreliable, especially in children. Furthermore, difficulty exists in defining signs and symptoms qualitatively.

Finally, the terms 'dysfunction' and 'parafunction' are often mixed up. Strictly defined, dysfunction is a partial disturbance, impairment or abnormality of the functioning of an organ, whereas parafunction is a disordered or perverted function, which can cause a dysfunction. This situation is made even more confusing by the fact that parafunctions are sometimes included in subjective symptoms and sometimes as clinical signs. In a critical review, Luther (1998) stated that more information with respect to TMD and malocclusion is needed. His request deserves attention for the diagnosis of the different malocclusions as well. So for example, a literature search on 'crossbite' will result in a malocclusion with different localization such as 'anterior', 'posterior', 'lateral', and even 'buccal' crossbite, each of them often in combination with another dental anomaly (Thilander and Bjerklin, 2012). To classify these different malocclusion types in the same category may explain the controversial opinions on its possible association with TMD, before as well as after an orthodontic treatment.

Due to such inaccuracy, related to the classification of the malocclusion and the concept of TMD, we cannot guarantee that our orthodontic patients will be free from possible adverse TMD. Thus, examination of the morphological malocclusions must be completed with a functional examination of the masticatory system before initiation of the orthodontic treatment, at the end of the treatment and preferably at post-retention period.

Conclusions

Application of a force on the crown of the tooth results in a tooth movement, which depends on type, magnitude, direction and duration of the force. The tissue response in this process is of fundamental significance in making the proper use of biomechanical principles to avoid adverse tissue reactions, such as root resorption and bone dehiscence.

Plaque accumulation around bands and brackets may cause gingival inflammation and retraction, and even demineralisation of the enamel surface, called white spot lesions (WSL). Thus, each patient has to follow a proper dental hygiene programme.

In a patient who is not allergic to nickel, the risk is virtually nonexistent to develop a nickel allergy because of the nickel-containing appliance. If some form of piercing is planned and orthodontic treatment is discussed, it is appropriate to carry out the orthodontic treatment first, since a slow and low concentration release of nickel ions from the orthodontic appliance means a tolerance of developing nickel allergy in the future.

Pain and discomfort are mainly reported during the first week after insertion of an orthodontic appliance. Pain scores overall peak between 12 hours and 3 days after insertion, and the scores return to baseline at day 7 and remain at baseline level throughout the whole treatment period.

From a general point of view, orthodontic therapy in children and adolescents is not a risk for the development of TMD.

REFERENCES

Aass, A.M. and Gjermo, P. (1992) Changes in radiographic bone level in orthodontically treated teenagers over a 4-year period. Community Dent Oral Epidemiol 20: 90–93.

Albander, J.M., Rise, J., Gjermo, P. and Johansen, J.R. (1986) Radiographic quantification of alveolar bone level changes: a 2-year longitudinal study in man. J Clin Periodontol 13: 195–200.

Altuna, G., Lewis, D.W., Chao, I. et al. (1991) A statistical assessment of orthodontic practices, product usage, and the development of skin lesions. Am J Orthod Dentofacial Orthop 100: 242–250.

Bergius, M., Kiliaridis, S. and Berggren, U. (2000) Pain in orthodontics: a review and discussion of the literature. J Orofacial Orthop 61: 125–137.

Bondemark, L. (1998) Interdental bone changes after orthodontic treatment: a 5-year longitudinal study. Am J Orthod Dentofacial Orthop 114: 25–31.

Boyd, R. and Baumrind, S. (1992) Periodontal considerations in the use of bonds or bands on molars in adolescents and adults. Angle Orthod 62: 117–126.

Brudvik, P. and Rygh, P. (1994) Root resorption beneath the main hyalinised zone. Eur J Orthod 16: 249–263.

Brudvik, P. and Rygh, P. (1995) Transition and determinants of orthodontic root resorption – repair sequence. Eur J Orthod 17: 177–188.

Chapman, J.A., Roberts, W.E., Eckert, G.J. *et al.* (2010) Risk factors for incidence and severity of white spot lesions during treatment with fixed orthodontic appliances. Am J Orthod Dentofacial Orthop 138: 188–194.

Derks, A., Katsaros, C., Frencken, J.E. *et al.* (2004) Caries-inhibiting effect of preventive measures during orthodontic treatment with fixed appliances. A systematic review. Caries Res 38: 413–420.

Dibbets, J. and van der Wehle, L. (1987) Orthodontic treatment in relation to symptoms attributed to dysfunction of the temporomandibilar joint. A 10-year report of the University of Gronningen study. Am J Orthod Dentofacial Orthop 91: 193–199.

Egermark, I. and Thilander, B. (1992) Craniomandibular disorders with special reference to orthodontic treatment: an evaluation from childhood to adulthood. Am J Orthod Dentofacial Orthop 101: 28–34.

Ericsson, I., Thilander, B., Lindhe, J, and Okamoto, H. (1977) The effect of orthodontic tilting movements on the periodontal tissues of infected and non-infected dentitions in dogs. J Clin Periodontol 4: 278–293.

Feasby, W.H., Ecclestone, E.R. and Grainger, R.M. (1988) Nickel sensitivity in pediatric dental patients. Pediatr Dent 10: 127–129.

Feldmann, I., List, T. and Bondemark, L. (2012) Orthodontic anchoring techniques and its influences on pain, discomfort, and jaw function – a randomized controlled trial. Eur J Orthod 34: 102–108.

Fors, R., Stenberg, B., Stenlund, H. *et al.* (2012) Nickel allergy in relation to piercing and orthodontic appliances – a population study. Contact Dermatitis 67: 342–350.

Flyvholm, M.A., Nielsen, G.D. and Andersen, A. (1984) Nickel content of food and estimation of dietary intake. Z Lebensm Unters Forsch 179: 427–431.

Henrikson, T. (1999) Temporomandibular disorders and mandibular function in relation to Class II malocclusion and orthodontic treatment. A controlled, prospective and longitudinal study. Swed Dent J Suppl 134: 1–144.

Hollender, L., Rönnerman, A. and Thilander, B. (1980) Root resorption, marginal bone support and clinical crown length in orthodontically treated patients. Eur J Orthod 2: 197–205.

Jacobsen, N. and Hensten-Pettersen, A. (2003) Changes in occupational health problems and adverse patient reactions in orthodontics from 1987 to 2000. Eur J Orthod 25: 591–598.

Johal, A., Fleming, P.S. and Al Jawad, F.A. (2014) A prospective longitudinal controlled assessment of pain experience and oral health-related quality of life in adolescents undergoing fixed appliance treatment. Orthod Craniofacial Res 17: 178–186.

Kerosuo, H., Kullaa, A., Kerosuo, E. *et al.* (1996) Nickel allergy in adolescents in relation to orthodontic treatment and piercing of ears. Am J Orthod Dentofacial Orthop 109: 148–154.

Ketcham, A.H. (1929) A progress report of an investigation of apical root resorption of vital permanent teeth. Int J Orthod 15: 310–328.

Kjaer, I. (1995) Morphological characteristics of dentitions developing excessive root resorption during orthodontic treatment. Eur J Orthod 17: 25–34.

Kurol, J., Owman-Moll, P. and Lundgren D (1996) Time-related root resorption after application of a controlled continuous orthodontic force. Am J Orthod Dentofacial Orthop 110: 303–310.

Kvam, E. (1972) Scanning electron microscopy of tissue changes on the pressure surface of human premolars following tooth movement. Scand J Dent Res 80: 357–368.

Levander, E. and Malmgren, O. (1988) Evaluation of the risk of root resorption during orthodontic treatment: a study of upper incisors. Eur J Orthod 10: 30–38.

Lund, H., Gröndahl, K., Hansen, K. *et al.* (2012) Apical root resorption during orthodontic treatment. A prospective study using cone beam CT. Angle Orthod 82: 480–487.

Luther, F. (1998) Orthodontics and the temporomandibular joint: where are we now? Part 2. Functional occlusion, mal-occlusion, and TMD. Angle Orthod 68: 305–318.

Sadowsky, C. and Polsen, A. (1984) Temporomandibular disorders and functional occlusion after orthodontic treatment: results of two long-term studies. Am J Orthod 86: 386–390.

Scheurer, P.A., Firestone, A.R. and Burgin, W.B. (1996) Perception of pain as a result of orthodontic treatment with fixed appliances. Eur J Orthod 18: 349–357.

Sonesson, M., Twetman, S. and Bondemark, L. (2014) Effectiveness of high-fluoride toothpaste on enamel demineralization during orthodontic treatment – a multi-centre randomized controlled trial. Eur J Orthod 36: 678–682.

Tanaka, T., Marioka, T., Ayasaka, N. *et al.* (1990) Endocytosis in odontoclasts and osteoclasts using microperoxidase as a tracer. J Dent Res 69: 883–889.

Thilander, B. and Bjerklin, K. (2012) Posterior crossbite and temporo-mandibular disorders (TMDs): need for orthodontic treatment? Eur J Orthod 34: 667–673.

Vukovich, M.E., Wood, D.P. and Daley, T.D. (1991) Heat generated by grinding during removal of ceramic brackets. Am J Orthod Dentofacial Orthop 99: 505–512.

Wiedel, A.P. and Bondemark, L. (2016) A randomized controlled trial of self-perceived pain, discomfort, and impairment of jaw function in children undergoing orthodontic treatment with fixed or removable appliances. Angle Orthod 86: 324–330.

Weltman, B., Vig, K.W.L., Fields, H.W. *et al.* (2010) Root resorption associated with orthodontic tooth movement: a systematic review. Am J Orthod Dentofacial Orthop 137: 462–476.

Wennström, J., Lindhe, J., Sinclair, F. *et al.* (1987) Some periodontal tissue reactions to orthodontic movement in monkeys. J Clin Periodontol 14: 121–129.

CHAPTER 12

Retention and post-retention outcome

Birgit Thilander, Krister Bjerklin and Lars Bondemark

Key topics

- Retention
- The concept relapse
- Post-retention outcome

Learning objectives

- To understand the definition 'relapse'
- To describe the biological process during the relapse period
- To discuss the length of the retention period
- To understand and describe possible changes during the post-retention period

Essential Orthodontics, First Edition. Birgit Thilander, Krister Bjerklin and Lars Bondemark.
© 2018 John Wiley & Sons Ltd. Published 2018 by John Wiley & Sons Ltd.

Introduction

The orthodontic correction in growing children is just an event during a period of growth and development in the patient's life. Although the interrelation between the teeth becomes established in childhood, continuous small changes occur throughout life, and the same is true for the craniofacial morphology, as described in Chapter 3. In this dynamic environment of continuing skeletal changes, functional demands and compensatory adaptations of the dentition, the orthodontic treatment is performed.

After withdrawal of the orthodontic forces, the retention period will take over. Orthodontic correction will remain stable if the teeth are aligned into a normal occlusion and provided with adequate retention. Moreover, the patient expects that the orthodontist shall finish the treatment period with an optimal result and stability that will last for years. However, every orthodontist knows that some patients will experience a tendency for the teeth to return to their original position, even after years of retention, a phenomenon described as relapse.

Retention

After the active orthodontic correction, the real problem will arise, i.e. how to retain and for how long, to obtain a stable result. Many different removable or fixed retainers have been used and each of them has both advantages and disadvantages. Bonded retainers in the incisor region of the mandible or maxilla are an often-used choice as they are independent of cooperation. The retainers can be bonded to the canines only, to the incisors and canines, or to incisors only (Figure 12.1). Also, removable retainers in the maxilla like a Jensen retainer (Figure 12.2), a vacuum formed splint (Essix stent) (Figure 12.3), a Hawley plate or some of its many modifications can be used (Shawesh *et al.*, 2010; Thickett and Power, 2010).

A systematic review of the stability and side effects of orthodontic retainers (Bondemark *et al.*, 2007) has shown low quality of evidence between fixed and removable retainers as regards stability, as well as presence of calculus or dental caries prevalence between the different types of retainers. Most often the choice of retention

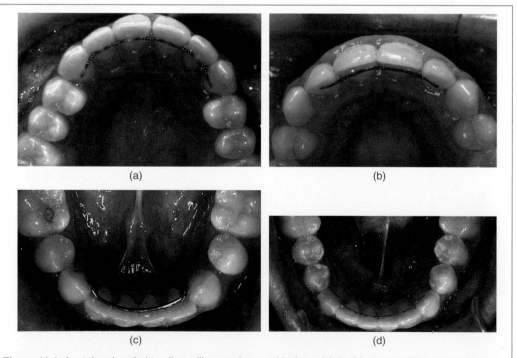

(a)

(b)

(c)

(d)

Figure 12.1 A retainer bonded to all maxillary canines and incisors (a). In (b), the maxillary retainer is bonded to the four incisors. In (c), a canine-to-canine is inserted and bonded to the mandibular canines only, while in (d), the retainer is bonded to both mandibular canines and all incisors.

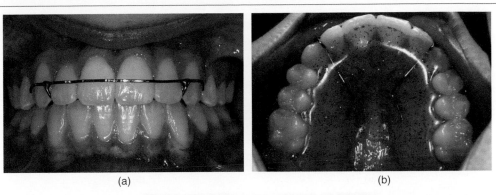

Figure 12.2 The Jensen retainer with its typical labial arch wire for stabilization of the maxillary incisors (a), and in (b), the occlusal view of the retainer.

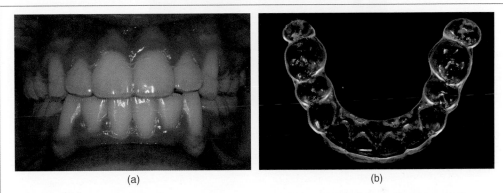

Figure 12.3 The Essix retainer is a vacuum-formed stent that is entirely made of transparent plastic that fits over all or mostly all teeth in the jaw (a), and the occlusal view of the retainer (b).

device depends on individual factors such as type of the initial malocclusion and expected patient cooperation.

The length of the retention period is controversial. Some recommend 2 to 5 years, whereas others have suggested a minimum of 10 years or longer. Of importance to remember is that if an undesirable growth pattern is treated only by compensations in the dentoalveolar system, subsequent post-treatment growth may upset a result that looks good when the patient is young.

The concept relapse

Type of retainer and length of retention period are connected to relapse, a concept that has been discussed for years and still leaves many questions unanswered. Many theories have been proposed as to the aetiology of relapse,

and many treatment and retention strategies have been recommended to minimise undesirable post-treatment changes. In general, an orthodontic tooth movement which is opposed to the direction of functional tooth migration is more liable to relapse than one in which the direction corresponds. Teeth that have been rotated tend to return to their former position. Supra-alveolar fibres are under tension by tooth rotation. Cutting through these fibres (fibretomy) can reduce the relapse of rotated maxillary incisors (Edwards, 1970).

A relapse from an orthodontic point of view is defined as 'a return towards pre-treatment conditions', and hence is an event of periodontal tissue reaction or dentofacial developmental changes. A general widening of the dental arches, particularly in the mandibular incisor area, will be prone to relapse, even after years of retention. In addition, orthodontic relapse

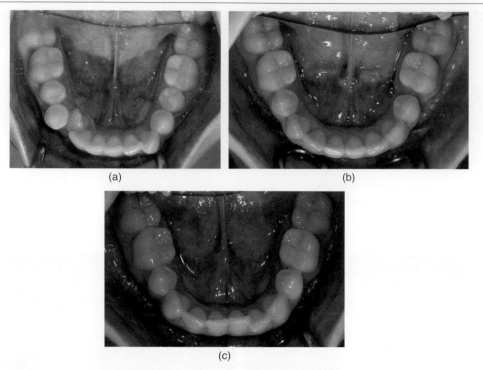

(a)

(b)

(c)

Figure 12.4 In (a), before treatment, and in (b), after treatment. In (c), relapse of one of the mandibular incisors.

of incisors is the real complaint for the patients due to the aesthetic aspects (Figure 12.4), while possible relapse of skeletal malocclusion ('orthopaedic relapse') seems to be of less importance.

As stated in Chapter 10, condyles and sutures respond to orthopaedic forces by changing the growth direction, and when the force is discontinued, the individual growth pattern takes over. If this is a 'relapse', it should be questioned about its definition 'return to the original position'. This assertion is verified by a longitudinal follow-up study with the Herbst appliance (Pancherz *et al.*, 2015), in which the importance of late adult facial growth changes must be considered in dentofacial orthopaedics with respect to treatment timing, post-treatment retention and relapse. Thus, the orthopaedic relapse is an indication that the individual growth pattern takes over again during the post-treatment period.

Experimental studies have shown that the tooth will return to its former position if the orthodontically moved tooth is not retained to allow synchronous remodelling of the tooth-supporting tissues (Reitan, 1967). The most persistent relapse tendency is caused by the structures related to the marginal third of the root, whereas little relapse tendency exists in the area adjacent to the middle and apical root, as shown in an experimental tipped incisor in the dog over a period of 40 days. Some relapse was noted already after 2 hours, partly caused by the tooth regaining a more upright position within the periodontal space. Still more relapse occurred on the following 3 days for a total of about 1.5 mm, and after this the tooth came to a standstill during some days, caused by hyalinisation on the former tension side, which due to the relapse had been transformed into a pressure side. Fibre contraction seems to be strong enough to produce hyalinisation. After elimination of the hyalinised tissue, the tooth continued to relapse. A similar pattern was observed in children after tipping teeth without a subsequent retention. The documentation calls for immediate insertion of a retention device because of this rapid relapse after orthodontic tooth movement. Furthermore, it warrants the following reminder in preprosthetic orthodontics; a temporary bridge must be inserted after preparation of teeth for fixed prosthodontic restorations to avoid such a rapid orthodontic relapse.

The tissue reactions in the gingiva differ from those in the periodontal ligament (PDL) and are of different importance for the stability of the new position of the orthodontically moved tooth. The various fibre groups also respond differently to the remodelling process. Furthermore, both supra-alveolar and periodontal tissues develop during the eruption of teeth, which explains the greater stability of teeth that are guided during the eruptive period, compared with teeth that are moved after having reached occlusion. This explains the greater stability of teeth that are guided passively into position during the eruptive period compared with teeth that are moved orthodontically after having reached occlusal stability. According to Reitan (1967), there will be little or no relapse following orthodontic movement of an erupting tooth, since its supporting tissues are in a proliferation stage. New fibres will be formed as the root develops, and these new fibres will assist in maintaining the new tooth position.

Unlike the PDL, the supra-alveolar fibres are not anchored in a bony wall that can be readily remodelled, where they have less chance of being reorganised, as the collagen turnover in PDL is five times as high as in the attached gingiva (Svoboda *et al.*, 1981). It is generally agreed that the collagen turnover in the PDL is fastest in the apical region of the root and slowest in the cervical region. Furthermore, there is a decrease in collagen turnover in all regions with age (Hennemann *et al.*, 2012). Among the gingival fibres, the trans-septal fibres show the fastest turnover rate, as fast as in the PDL (Redlich *et al.*, 1999).

The slower turnover of the gingival fibres easily explains why such fibres are seen stretched and un-remodelled as long as 232 days after experimental rotation (Reitan 1959). The stretched fibre bundles on the tension side tend to become relaxed and rearranged according to the physiologic movement of the tooth. The reason for this slow remodelling probably is related to the quality of fibre groups, whose main function is to maintain tooth position and interproximal contact.

The trans-septal fibre system stabilises teeth against separating forces and may maintain the contacts of adjacent teeth in a state of compression. Removal of proximal tooth contact will allow the trans-septal fibre system to contract and so cause an approximation of the adjacent teeth. This interproximal force is increased after occlusal loading (Southard *et al.*, 1992) and it appears that the periodontium itself may be linked to post-treatment relapse.

Apart from the trans-septal and dentoperiosteal fibres of the gingiva, the fibrils connecting heavy maxillary frenulum attachment to the alveolar process need a very long period of remodelling. In addition, the presence of elastic and elastic-like fibres (oxytalan) in the gingiva has been suggested to play a role in the relapse tendency (Edwards, 1988). However, according to Sims (1976) and Jonas and Riede (1980), the oxytalan fibres are not stretched by orthodontic tooth movement and consequently cannot contribute to relapse. Hence, it is important to use a retention appliance as long as the remodelling process takes place, and by that avoid a 'rapid relapse'.

Post-retention period

The long-term effect of orthodontic treatment is of utmost importance for the patient, who takes it for granted that the orthodontic active treatment followed by the retention period shall result in a permanent ideal dental occlusion. However, studies on the long-term effect of orthodontic tooth movement have shown that 40 to 90% of the patients have dental irregularities 10 to 20 years' post-treatment, changes showing large individual and unpredictable variations (Little *et al.*, 1988; Sadowsky *et al.*, 1994; Kahl-Nieke *et al.*, 1995; Al Yami *et al.*, 1999; Schütz-Fransson *et al.*, 2016).

It is important to evaluate the degree of this relapse and to decide how to proceed in a possible re-treatment dilemma, while there is need for indexes. The Peer Assessment Rating (PAR) index (Richmond *et al.*, 1992) is used both as a self-evaluation instrument for the orthodontist to measure his/her own quality, and as a measuring tool to assess overall quality

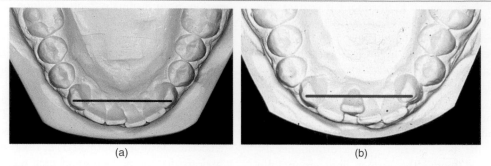

Figure 12.5 In (a), a male 16 years of age with Class I occlusion, acceptable and small crowding of mandibular incisors, congenitally missing 3rd molars and no treatment needed. In (b), the same subject at 31 years of age and still Class I occlusion but now high demand for orthodontic treatment because of severe crowded mandibular incisors. Note also the diminished intercanine width of approximately 2 mm that have arisen between 16 and 31 years of age (black line versus blue line).

in larger samples. This method has its limitations due to the task of the clinician to decide whether the post-treatment changes are acceptable or not, a highly subjective judgement (Al Yami *et al.*, 1998). The irregularity index (the sum of the labial-lingual overlap of the six mandibular incisors) by Little (1975) is limited to the mandibular incisor region and does not always give a valid estimate of the space deficit.

Many causative factors to the post-retention 'relapse' have been discussed in the literature, accompanied by cause-and-effect conclusions for clinical guidelines. Eruption of the third molars, position of the mandibular incisors, the mandibular growth-rotation, and oral habits are causative factors, often debated. Contradictory results have been presented, and the large individual outcome has been stressed. Most studies indicate that it is difficult or impossible to point out a single factor, and instead it seems to be a multifactorial problem. Post-orthodontic cranial changes may be the most significant causative factors (Nanda and Nanda, 1992; Harris *et al.*, 1999; Ormiston *et al.*, 2005; Thilander *et al.*, 2005; Bondevik, 2012), but also post-retention tooth changes are also of utmost importance for this 'relapse' (Little *et al.*, 1988; De la Cruz *et al*, 1995; Gardner *et al.*, 1998). However, the post-retention changes can be difficult to distinguish from the ageing changes in the individual. This statement is in accordance with the findings by Vaden *et al.* (1997), who showed that the rate of post-retention changes decreased with time, and clinical follow-up studies in patients not orthodontically

treated (Sinclair and Little, 1983; Richardson, 1995; Bishara *et al.*, 1998; Bondevik, 1998; Henrikson *et al.*, 2001; Thilander, 2009; Jonsson *et al.*, 2010; Tsiopas *et al.*, 2013).

Analysis of orthodontically and non-orthodontically treated cases in follow-up studies is of importance to learn more about post-retention development versus relapse. So, for example, a longitudinal study of subjects with well-shaped dental arches and normal occlusion ('ideal cases'), not orthodontically treated, clearly showed the dentofacial changes from early childhood into adolescence, young adulthood and late adulthood, changes that are a gradual process that has to be taken into consideration in orthodontic treatment. Length, depth and width of the dental arches showed continuous changes of importance for the post-retention stability, which may explain why 12 of the 30 'ideal' subjects, examined at adult ages, showed incisor crowding of different degrees (Figure 12.5), even in cases with congenitally missing third molars.

Conclusions

The continuous dentoalveolar changes, known as physiological tooth migration, should be distinguished from orthodontic relapse, and the occlusion is to be regarded as a dynamic rather than a static interrelation between facial structures. However, relapse after orthodontic treatment and the natural physiological changes are difficult to predict on an individual basis.

It can be asked whether it is realistic to expect long-term stability after orthodontic treatment but of course, life-long retention can be advocated, but in such cases, the retention will counteract the normal physiological changes. Thus, the length of the retention period to avoid 'relapse' seems to be a basis for future research and discussions among orthodontists.

REFERENCES

Al Yami, E., Kuijpers-Jagtman, A.M. and van't Hof, M. (1998). Assessment of biological changes in a nonorthodontic sample using the PAR index. Am J Orthod Dentofacial Orthop 114: 224–228.

Al Yami, E., Kuijpers-Jagtman, A.M. and van't Hof, M. (1999). Stability of orthodontic treatment outcome: follow-up until 10 years postretention. Am J Orthod Dentofacial Orthop 115: 300–304.

Bishara, S., Jacobsen, J., Treder, I. *et al.* (1998) Arch length changes from 6 weeks to 45 years. Angle Orthod 68: 69–74.

Bondemark, L., Holm, A.K., Hansen, K. *et al.* (2007) Long-term stability of orthodontic treatment and patient satisfaction. A systematic review. Angle Orthod 77: 181–191.

Bondevik, O. (1998) Changes in occlusion between 23 and 34 years. Angle Orthod 68: 75–80.

Bondevik, O. (2012) Dentofacial changes in adults: a longitudinal chephalometric study in 22–33 and 33–43 years olds. J Orofacial Orthop 73: 277–288.

De La Cruz, A., Sampson, P., Little, R.M. *et al.* (1995) Long-term changes in arch form after orthodontic treatment and retention. Am J Orthod Dentofacial Orthop 107: 518–530.

Edwards, J.G. (1970) A surgical procedure to eliminate rotational relapse. Am J Orthod 57: 35–46.

Edwards, J.G. (1988) A long-term prospective evaluation of the circumferential supracrestal fiberotomy in alleviating orthodontic relapse. Am J Orthod Dentofacial Orthop 93: 380–387.

Gardner, R., Harris, E. and Vaden, J. (1998) Postorthodontic dental changes: a longitudinal study. Am J Orthod Dentofacial Orthop 114: 581–586.

Harris, E., Gardner, R., and Vaden, J. (1999) A longitudinal cephalometric study of postorthodontic craniofacial changes. Am J Orthod Dentofacial Orthop 115: 77–82.

Henneman, S., Reijers, R., Maltha, J. and Von den Hoff, J. (2012) Local variations in turnover of periodontal collagen fibres in rats. J Periodontal Res 47: 383–388.

Henrikson, J., Persson, M. and Thilander, B. (2001) Long-term stability of dental arch form in normal occlusion from 13 to 31 years of age. Eur J Orthod 23: 51–61.

Jonas, I. and Riede, U. (1980) Reaction of oxytalan fibres in human periodontium to mechanical stress. A combined histochemical and morphometric analysis. J Histochem Cytochem 28: 211–216.

Jonsson, T., Karlsson, K.O., Ragnarsson, B. *et al.* (2010) Long-term development of malocclusion traits in orthodontically treated and untreated subjects. Am J Orthod Dentofacial Orthop 138: 277–284.

Kahl-Nieke, B., Fischbach, H. and Schwarze, C. (1995) Post-retention crowding and incisor irregularity: a long-term follow-up evaluation of stability and relapse. Br J Orthod 22: 249–257.

Little, R.M. (1975) The irregularity index: a quantitative score of mandibular anterior alignment. Am J Orthod 68: 554–563.

Little, R.M., Riedel, R.A. and Årtun, J. (1988) An evaluation of changes in mandibular anterior alignment from 10 to 20 years postretention. Am J Orthod Dentofacial Orthop 93: 425–428.

Nanda, R.S. and Nanda, S.K. (1992) Considerations of dentofacial growth in long-term retention and stability: is active retention needed? Am J Orthod Dentofacial Orthop 101: 297–302.

Ormiston, J., Huang, G., Little, R.M. *et al.* (2005) Retrospective analysis of long-term stable and unstable orthodontic treatment outcomes. Am J Orthod Dentofacial Orthop 128: 568–574.

Pancherz, H., Bjerklin, K. and Hashemi, K. (2015) Late adult skeletofacial growth after adolescent Herbst therapy: A 32-year longitudinal follow-up study. Am J Orthod Dentofacial Orthop 147: 19–28.

Redlich, M., Shoshan, S. and Palmon, A. (1999) Gingival response to orthodontic force. Am J Orthod Dentofacial Orthop 116: 152–158.

Reitan, K. (1959) Tissue rearrangement during retention of orthodontically rotated teeth. Angle Orthod 29: 105–113.

Reitan, K. (1967) Clinical and histologic observations on tooth movement during and after orthodontic treatment. Am J Orthod 53: 721–745.

Richardson, M.E. (1995) Late lower arch crowding: the role of the transverse dimension. Am J Orthod Dentofacial Orthop 107: 613–617.

Richmond, S., Shaw, W., O'Brien, K. *et al.* (1992) The development of the PAR (Peer Assessment Rating) index: reliability and validity. Eur J Orthod 14: 125–139.

Sadowsky, C., Schneider, B., BeCole, E. *et al.* (1994) Long-term stability after orthodontic treatment: nonextraction with prolonged retention. Am J Orthod Dentofacial Orthop 106: 243–249.

Shawesh, M., Bhatti, B., Usman, T. *et al.* (2010) Hawley retainers full- or part-time? Eur J Orthod 32: 165–170.

Sims, M. (1976) Reconstitution of the human oxytalan system during orthodontic tooth movement. Am J Orthod 70: 38–58.

Sinclair, P.M. and Little, R.M. (1983) Maturation of untreated normal occlusions. Am J Orthod 83: 114–123.

Southard, T., Southard, K. and Tolley, E. (1992) Periodontal force: a potential cause of relapse. Am J Orthod Dentofacial Orthop 101: 221–227.

Svoboda, E., Shiga, A., and Deporter, D. (1981) A stereologic analysis of collagen phagocytosis by fibroblasts in three soft connective tissues with differing rates of collagen turnover. Anat Rec 199: 473–480.

Schütz-Fransson, U., Lindsten, R., Bjerklin, K. *et al.* (2016) Twelve-year follow-up of mandibular incisor stability: comparison between two bonded lingual orthodontic retainers. Angle Orthod. August 23. [Epub ahead of print].

Thickett, E. and Power, S. (2010) A randomised clinical trial of thermoplastic retainer wear. Eur J Orthod 32: 1–5.

Thilander, B., Persson, M. and Adolfsson, U. (2005) Roentgen-cephalometric standards for a Swedish population. A longitudinal study between the ages of 5 and 31 years of age. Eur J Orthod 27: 370–389.

Thilander, B. (2009) Dentoalveolar development in subjects with normal occlusion. A longitudinal study between the ages of 5 and 31 years. Eur J Orthod 31: 109–120.

Tsiopas, N., Nilner, M., Bondemark, L. *et al.* (2013) A 40 years follow-up of dental arch dimensions and incisor irregularity in adults. Eur J Orthod 35: 230–235.

Vaden, J., Harris, E. and Gardner, R. (1997) Relapse revisited. Am J Orthod Dentofacial Orthops 111: 543–553.

Index

Essential Orthodontics, First Edition. Birgit Thilander, Krister Bjerklin and Lars Bondemark.
© 2018 John Wiley & Sons Ltd. Published 2018 by John Wiley & Sons Ltd.